REDEEMED SEXUALITY

A Guide to Sexuality for Christian Singles, Campus Students, Teens and Parents

Tim Konzen and Dr. Jennifer Konzen

ELM HILL

A Division of
HarperCollins Christian Publishing

www.elmhillbooks.com

Redeemed Sexuality
A Guide to Sexuality for Christian Singles,
Campus Students, Teens and Parents

Published in Nashville, Tennessee, by Elm Hill, an imprint of Thomas Nelson. Elm Hill and Thomas Nelson are registered trademarks of HarperCollins Christian Publishing, Inc.

Content Editor: Robin Weidner

Cover Design by Beth Weeks, SDSU School of Art & Design Managing Editor and Layout Designer: Beth Lottig

Elm Hill titles may be purchased in bulk for educational, business, fund-raising, or sales promotional use. For information, please e-mail SpecialMarkets@ ThomasNelson.com.

Scripture taken from the HOLY BIBLE, NEW INTERNATIONAL VERSION˙ NIV˙ Copyright © 1973, 1978, 1984, 2011 by Biblica, Inc.˙ Used by permission. All rights reserved worldwide.

Library of Congress Cataloging-in-Publication Data

Pre-Launch ISBN 978-1-595559517

Library of Congress Control Number: 2018939114

ISBN 978-1-595543516
ISBN 978-1-595556066 (eBook)

ACKNOWLEDGMENTS

Redeemed Sexuality came about because it was requested. At the time of the writing of this book, we have two high school students and two college students. Their friends are in our home all the time, and the teen and campus students either hang out, eat, or fellowship at our home regularly. When some of them began to hear about our book for married couples, The Art of Intimate Marriage, the question was spoken over and over, "Do you have a book for singles?" So our real gratitude goes to those singles and students who let their needs be known and who, like the disciples who said, "Teach us to pray," they asked, "Teach us about sex." Parents and those who lead ministries for teens, campus students, and singles have asked the same thing. We get calls from leaders and parents with questions on how to guide these young men and women in their sexual lives. Our thanks especially go to Cindi Whitcomb and Lisa Payne of the Los Angeles church for saying, "Help!" Those many requests for help became this book.

We have had some incredible couples in our lives who have helped us raise and love our own children. Words cannot express our gratitude for those who have helped us through these years. Some of you have discipled us, some of you have advised us from across many miles, and some of you have been dear friends walking this road with us. Thank you to Guillermo and Terry Adame, Ron and Linda Brumley, Ray and

Janet Schalk, Paul and Kerry Schultz, Guy and Cathy Hammond, and Sheridan and Debbie Wright.

The production of this work has been possible because of some truly talented and generous people. There have been some persevering readers, editors, and designers whose input and encouragement has been invaluable. We especially want to thank Linda Brumley, Austin Boyd, Lanie Bennaton, and our editors, Beth Lottig and Robin Weidner, for reading many words and giving much needed input about those words. Thank you to Selena Idioma for the advanced readers copy book cover and the inspiration for the final cover. The beauty of this book is the result of two Beths, Beth Lottig and Beth Weeks. Thank you Beth Weeks for your beautiful interior and cover design and thank you Beth Lottig for being at the helm. You are a joy to work with. Also, for the many years of training Jennifer has received in sexuality, thank you Debra Taylor and Dr. Irwin Goldstein.

Our time with our kids is like an island in the ocean and an oasis in the desert. They have also put up with all the crazy material on our book shelves, on the table, next to the chair, and on the floor. You guys bring us so much joy. Our hope is that each of you will experience the same fun and fulfillment your parents have found in living out their marriage to glorify God. We love being your parents.

Putting this together, with all the many scriptures involved, has been a continual reminder of how wonderful it is to have God hold our hands on this journey. We are grateful that God hears our prayers and walks with us through the rivers and through the fire.

In gratitude,
Tim and Jennifer

CONTENTS

INTRODUCTION

Parental Advisory: If you are thinking of having your teen read this book, it's best if that happens after you have already had a healthy, open conversation about sex with them. We generally recommend that the "how babies are made" conversation starts in the early grade school years (i.e., first grade or so), with many regular times of follow-up afterwards. If that has not happened with your children, it's not too late. You can do it now. You will find direction for that in the last section of this book. If you do not initiate these types of conversations, someone else will. They have most likely already received sexual information via the Internet, on their school campus, or in conversations between friends. We recommend you read this book together with your child. Read a chapter and then talk about it. Read another and then talk some more.

From the beginning of this book, we will be using sexually explicit terms. If you are giving this to your teen to read or are unsure if they are ready to read this with you, seek counsel. Even in the most spiritual family, sexual topics can be sensitive and cause reactions. As you, the parent, become more comfortable, your teen will also probably relax. It can help to remind them (and yourself) that God created sex. Our bodies are sexual. We desperately need to be able to discuss this topic openly, honestly, respectfully, wisely, and biblically. With that in mind, let us continue.

When we think about sex, we often think about intercourse. When we picture what sex is, we picture two bodies engaged in the act of sex. Yet sex is so much more than that. It is more than just the experience of orgasm. It is more than the sexual parts of our bodies (our genitals). Our sexuality has the potential of being an amazing door through which we come to a deeper understanding of God. And this does not mean that the act of intercourse is that door, though it may be a part of it. Sex encompasses much more than the act of intercourse. In fact, there are people who live their whole lives without intercourse or orgasm. And yet those people are sexual. God created us male and female. Everyone born in this act of creation is a sexual creature. How someone lives out their sexuality, how someone experiences sexuality, is uniquely individual for each person. When God created us, when He created us as sexual beings, His creation was that of a master artist. We are wonderfully and fearfully made (Psalm 139:14). It is so vital that we discover both the artwork and the artist.

The master artist took some time to detail His plan for sexuality. The Bible is the only world religion text that has an entire book devoted to sex. When we look deeply at the descriptions of the sensual relationship between the Beloved and the Lover in Song of Songs, we find a beautiful, romantic, and erotic picture of what God intends for marriage. It is poetic. It is art. God intended for sex to be good, and when someone allows God to guide them in how they engage in sex, sex can bring wonder and joy. The words God uses to describe the act of sex are passion, burning, honor, pleasing, satisfying, and intoxicating. God's description of martial sexuality is very positive.

However, sex, and all it entails, can also be a source of great pain, confusion, frustration, sorrow, and grief. This is especially true in how we involve ourselves in erotic sexuality. Erotic sexuality is our sexual thoughts, feelings, and desires and the physical ways we express them, such as fantasizing, sexual communication, viewing and listening to sexual material, self-touch/masturbation, mutual sexual touch to orgasm, and intercourse, etc. There are so many ways mankind can sin against one another (i.e., lying, fits of rage, being arrogant with one another, being selfish, unkind, or unloving, etc.), and each of the wounds from these kinds of sin can be difficult in unique ways.

Sexual wounds, however, are some of the most painful and the most difficult to heal. Those wounds can come from the choices we make, from the things that others do against us, and from the ways in which Satan has inundated the world with a tsunami of destructive words and images about sex.

The Scriptures teach that when sexual sin occurs, there is a unique impact on the person. "All other sins a person commits are outside the body, but whoever sins sexually, sins against their own body" (1 Corinthians 6:18). "The body, however, is not meant for sexual immorality but for the Lord, and the Lord for the body" (1 Corinthians 6:13).

The body is not meant for sexual immorality. What a simple and profound statement. Sexual sin affects our bodies and souls. This happens whether someone violates us physically, verbally, or sexually, or whether we violate our own dignity by seeking gratification outside of God's plan.

So how can we reconcile God's intricate and amazing plan for sexuality with the devastation that sex outside of His plan can cause? What exactly is redeemed sexuality?

What Is Redeemed Sexuality?

Webster's Dictionary defines redeemed as buying back or winning back; freeing something from distress, from harm or from captivity. Strong's concordance uses the word *exagorazo*, which means to fully buy out, to ransom. "Christ redeemed us from the curse of the law by becoming a curse for us" (Galatians 3:13). *Agorazo* means to buy. But the use of *exagorazo* means to go all out (*ex* is an intensifier), to do whatever it takes to buy something. That's what Jesus did. He went all out, giving everything He had, to redeem us, to buy us back, to bring us from the kingdom of darkness into His wonderful light.

We all need this redemption. The realm of sexual acts we might experience during this life could reflect both darkness and light. Though God is very positive about sex and intends our sexuality to be a source of great joy, there are so many things that can steal that joy. Within God's Word and within a life of following Jesus, we can experience redeemed sexuality. Imagine living out your sexuality as God intends, freed from any distress, captivity or harm Satan could inflict and seeing your sexuality instead as a joy and blessing (Galatians 3:14). One goal of this book is to answer the question, "What is God's plan for sex?" I mean, come on, when you see what the sexual genitals look like, you might think, "Really God, what is all that about?" A dear friend of ours once said that when she gets to heaven, one question she's going to ask God is why exactly He made genitals look as they do. They are a bit on the bizarre side when you really look at them. It can make us wonder—beyond the whole "be fruitful and increase in number" (Genesis 1:28) reproductive purpose of sex—what exactly does God want us to do with these parts of our bodies?

Another goal of this book is to specifically look at and come to an understanding of God's plan for sex for those who are not married—whether teens, college students, single, working professionals, or those who have once been married. We tend to think that discussions about sex are only for those who are married. That is actually a bit goofy when you think about it, as if the only time someone feels sexual or is a sexual person is when they are married. Our final goal is to give parents confidence in how to talk with their children about sex. There are parents who have said to their children, "Sex is only for marriage. We'll talk about it then." Or, "Just don't do it!" The lack of talking openly, honestly, and genuinely to our children about sex opens the door to our children feeling like sex is taboo. They might think that any sexual feelings, experiences, and thoughts are abnormal, dirty, and wrong; therefore they feel shameful for having them. This does not set up a child for having a healthy sexual relationship with their spouse in the future. It is important to remember, if you, as the parent, are not the one to have those conversations with your child, someone else will. The kids at school, the Internet, TV shows and movies, and the jokes they hear will become their source of education about sex. How much more beneficial it would be to hear about it from their parents who love them and desire to direct them into an understanding of the amazing God that created their amazing bodies.

So walk with us as we explore God's plan for sex and how to talk openly, genuinely, and honestly about the wonder of God's creation in all its glory.

So Who Are We?

From Tim: Jennifer's got a number of impressive credentials, and this isn't just coming from a biased husband; she's amazing. She has a doctorate in psychology and is a licensed marriage and family therapist, a certified sex therapist, a nationally award-winning sex researcher,[1] a certified chemical dependency counselor, an international speaker, and a professor. And, oh yeah, she also has a bachelor of music in musical theater/vocal performance. She always jokes that her next book is going to be titled Sex, Drugs, and Show Tunes. But on top of that, or as she will tell you, more importantly, she is a disciple of Jesus, a wife (lucky me), and a mother of four children. Those are her favorite jobs.

From Jennifer: Tim has impressive credentials as well. Not only did he do an amazing job of living as a single disciple pursuing purity, he has done a wonderful job raising our four children and has also supported me in all the crazy adventures I've had in learning to help people. Through our years together, he's been a middle school ministry leader, a youth and family shepherd, a married ministry leader, a financial adviser to the ministry leadership, and a deacon of benevolence and worship. His integrity and hard work as a program manager and business owner make him a great provider. But it is his genuine love for God and his sincere determination to stay faithful to his commitment to God, to me, to his children, and to God's kingdom that I truly love, need, and admire.

I, Tim, was converted in the singles ministry and Jennifer was converted as a campus student. Together we have enjoyed twenty-four years of marriage and parenting. Like many of you, we have struggled to keep our lives pure from sexual sin and to live as God desires in our sexual lives, both before we married and as a married couple. There have been so many who have helped us along the way for whom we are very grateful. In a similar way, we hope we can be a source of help to you as we all pursue honoring God in how we live out our sexuality.

---

[1] It should be noted that some of the research reported in this book, including Jennifer's, is based on Western, white participants and may not be generalizable to everyone, especially those from different ethnic, socioeconomic, racial, cultural, or national origins.

SECTION ONE

GOD'S PLAN

CHAPTER 1

WHAT DOES THE BIBLE
SAY ABOUT SEX?

Don't do it until you're married. Sexual sin will send you to hell.
When you're married, it is your duty.
Sex is something you do not talk about.
Having sexual thoughts and feelings is wrong.

The words above are about the sum total of what most people think the Bible says about sex. And if you are unmarried, sex is not something you should ever talk about. End of discussion. However, in His Word, God addresses sexuality in an open, deep way.

Some of you may be eager to learn God's perspective on sex. You may wish you knew more about what the Bible teaches about sex and God's view of sexuality. Some of you may find the whole topic uncomfortable or embarrassing. For others, you have read books and gone to numerous classes at conferences where they talked about staying pure and holy, but you're still feeling like you haven't gotten the kind of help you need. You have heard lots of lessons about how sex should be great, but only in marriage. The lessons unmarried people often hear about sex include what clothes they shouldn't wear, what music they shouldn't listen to, and what movies they shouldn't watch, etc. You may have heard a surplus of specifics on how to stay pure, but you still don't feel like you know how to interact with this body God has given you with all its sexual feelings and thoughts.

Or you may feel like you have gotten pat answers to the very genuine questions and real challenges you have. You may have felt frustrated and hopeless, or that you should just avoid the topic altogether. You may be seriously working on overcoming a purity struggle. You may be single, or a teen or campus student, and long for more guidance on dating, masturbation, purity, or how far you should go with a boyfriend or girlfriend. Or you may be a parent feeling like you do not know where to begin teaching your children about sexuality or how to help them navigate their own pursuit of purity. For parents, this chapter might be more for you than your child, especially if your child is a young teen or preteen. Or you may be a youth or campus ministry worker looking for resources for yourself and others. The first place to start in helping others with their convictions and practices around sexuality is to make sure your own are solid.

This chapter does not include everything the Bible has to say about sex. You will find specific detail on other scriptural aspects of sexuality in other chapters. But first, let's consider an overarching view of sexuality in the Scriptures. How can we view sexuality in a way that is life-transforming? This may require you to reexamine your beliefs and come to a new understanding of the biblical view. As you take a deeper look at the Scriptures in the Bible on sex, our prayer is that you'll feel empowered to bring how you are living out your sexuality closer to what God intends.

Sexuality and God

One of the areas around sexuality that can be very confusing for Christians is how to fit God in the picture. For many of us, it seems that our thoughts about sexuality have little connection to our thoughts about God. Sex is over here on the far right, and God is over here on the far left, and they never interact. Even saying God and sex in the same sentence seems kind of inappropriate. This is even truer for the words sex and Christ. After all, Jesus never even had sex, so it seems so inappropriate or even sacrilegious to put sex and Christ in the same sentence, right? What do the two have to do with each other?

Yet that is not what we find in the Bible. Jesus is to be Lord over every area of our lives. God speaks to us in every area of our lives, and that includes sexuality. We do not have to divorce ourselves from God and Jesus when we are discussing sexual topics, and God does not intend for any married couple to put God in the corner while they are experiencing the full, sensual enjoyment that is possible during sex.

Before beginning to specialize in sexuality in her counseling practice, Jennifer took some extensive time to look up every scripture that referenced sex. It has been important to us that what we teach in this incredibly sensitive area be faithfully based on the Word of God. Whether you are single, a student, or married, this is our first recommendation. If you are a ministry leader wanting to help people in the area of sexuality, and you want to grow in your competence in working with sexuality, this is our first recommendation. Ground yourself in what the Scriptures say about sex. To help you, we have included quite a few scriptures throughout this book that you can compare to your view of sexuality.

There are many books out there in the Christian publishing industry about sexuality and purity for singles and teens. There are also different scripts for how to talk to your children about sex. Although there is some helpful information out there, it is important to take a very critical stance when reading them. Some of these books, though the motivation of the author(s) may be to help, contain some biblical, psychological, and physiological errors. Some of them come from a shaming perspective in order to convince people to remain pure. Others take stances that may be contrary to the heart of the Scriptures and the heart God has about sexuality. We need to filter everything we read through the lens of the Scriptures. In the same way, we hope you take a critical view of what will be shared here. Do your own searching of the Scriptures to discover God's plan.

In our work—both professionally and in the ministry—we have

found that there is usually a lot of learning and relearning that has to happen in order to grasp God's perspective on sexuality. People often have to work through false beliefs about sex as well as the incredible pain, frustration, confusion, and fear that can surround this area of life. Be a noble Berean (Acts 17:11) and look up the scriptures and spiritual principles found in this book so that you can feel confident, convinced in your own mind (Romans 14:5), of what the Scriptures teach.

A Biblical View of Sexuality

> "The language and imagery of sexuality are the most graphic and most powerful that the Bible uses to describe the relationship between God and his people—both positively (when we are faithful) and negatively (when we are not)."
>
> —PIPER AND TAYLOR, SEX AND THE SUPREMACY OF CHRIST[1]

One of our favorite books for helping people understand a biblical and spiritual view of sex is Sex and the Supremacy of Christ by Piper and Taylor. The authors have kindly given permission to briefly review these two major points from their book: "God has designed sexuality as a way to know Him fully," and "Knowing God guards and guides our sexuality." As you read on, watch for how God uses the language and imagery of sexuality to communicate with us and to help us know Him. Note how our knowledge of God protects and directs how we live out our sexuality. "God Has Designed Sexuality as a Way to Know Him More Fully." This idea is found in the first chapter of Piper and Taylor's book. Please take a moment now to read Ezekiel 16 and then Ezekiel 23. When God is speaking about the nation of Israel and their worship of other idols, He uses words and phrases such as "prostitute," "lavished your favors," "degraded your beauty," "offering your body with increasing promiscuity to anyone who passed by," "your young breasts were fondled," "genitals...like

---

[1] Content paraphrased from Sex and the Supremacy of Christ, edited by John Piper and Justin Taylor, © 2005. Used by permission of Crossway, a publishing ministry of Good News Publishers, Wheaton, IL 60187. www. crossway.org.

those of donkeys," and "emission, like that of horses." Why would God use such graphic sexual language? For some, reading this might make you feel uncomfortable or may even make you laugh. Is this really in the Scriptures? Yet God uses sexual language to describe the spiritual choices Israel made in idol worship. Let's explore this together.

One of the biggest fears that married and unmarried people share is of their spouse (or future spouse) being unfaithful. For married people who've been through this, the emotional pain still may haunt them. This fear can be especially strong for those who saw their parents be unfaithful in their marriage. Those who engage in intimate relationships before marriage and experience unfaithfulness or a break-up also feel this agonizing betrayal. When the person you are in love with betrays you in some way, or if they have sex with someone while you are in a relationship together, the level of betrayal is deep and painful. We have sat with many who have expressed the devastating pain of sexual betrayal in their relationships, of finding out that the one they love has intimately touched another man or woman. Though this is true in any relationship, at any level of commitment, this is especially painful when it occurs in marriage.

When God talks in Ezekiel 16 and 23 about the incredible pain of Israel's betrayal with idols, He uses the language of sexual betrayal and adultery. He talks about it by using the analogy of the physical, sexual body—words such as breasts, genitals, and emission. Why? Because He wants us to understand His pain when we choose to worship something other than Him, when we turn our backs on Him and His love for us ("you became mine" Ezekiel 16:8). Because we intuitively understand the pain of sexual betrayal, God uses these pictures and words to describe the pain of betrayal He feels when we commit spiritual adultery, or idolatry, against Him. God uses sexual language to communicate His heart, who He is, and how He feels. He does this so that we can understand His heart and come close to Him. He wants us to know Him deeply.

In a similar way, God often uses other physical realities to help us understand the spiritual. For instance, He uses:

- The beauty and power of His creation to show us His beauty and power (Romans 1:20, Psalms 19:1-3)
- The way we are created to help us understand His image (Genesis 1:27)
- The incarnation, Jesus taking on a physical body, to show us what God looks like in human form (John 1:14, Isaiah 9:6, John 14:9, Colossians 1:15)

God uses the physical to express the spiritual. So it makes sense that God uses the physical language of sexuality to tell us about Himself and to communicate to us.

Knowing God

"I know my sheep and my sheep know me, just as the Father knows me and I know the Father" (John 10:14). God knows us. Jesus knows us. Jesus knows God and God the Father knows Jesus. The word know here is *gnosko* in the Greek, which means firsthand knowledge through personal experience; to learn, to recognize, to perceive. Gnosko is used here to describe the depth to which God and Jesus know each other. Their relationship is the ultimate example of an intimate understanding of the other at an indescribably deep level. What is interesting is that gnosko is the same word used to describe the sexual interaction between Joseph and Mary. "He (Joseph) did not know (gnosko) her (Mary) until she gave birth to a son" (Matthew 1:25; parenthetical references added). Gnosko is not only used to describe how well Jesus knows us, and how well Jesus and God know each other, but it is also used to explain the depth to which Joseph and Mary knew each other sexually.

We see something very similar in the Hebrew language. "No longer will a man teach his neighbor... 'Know the Lord,' because they will all know me" (Jeremiah 31:34). The Hebrew word here for know is *yada*, meaning to know, acknowledge, and understand through all the senses. And guess what? We find it also in Genesis 4:1. "Adam knew (yada) his wife Eve." So in both the Greek and Hebrew, the word for know describes how God knows us, how we know Jesus the Shepherd, how Jesus knows God, and how God wants us to know Him. Yada is also used to describe the sexual relationship between Adam and Eve and between Joseph and Mary.

In many translations, the word know in Genesis 4 and Matthew 1 is no longer used and has been variously translated to say "lay with her," or "had relations with her." The latest translation of the NIV reads, "made love to." Because the meaning of words is so dependent on the context they are in, the use of gnosko in both of these contexts is not to say (in any weird way) that our relationship with God or the relationship between God and Jesus has a sexual expression. That is what the pagan world did with false gods through their temple worship with prostitutes. But understanding this does help to convey how God intends us to understand the sexual relationship. The depth of intimate knowledge between Jesus and God, the depth to which He knows us and wants us to know Him, is the depth of intimacy God intends for those who are in a marital sexual relationship—a deep emotional, spiritual, and physical intimacy. These are the words God uses to describe sex.

This puts the importance of sexuality on a whole different level. John 17:3 says, "This is eternal life, that they know (gnosko) you, the only true God, and Jesus Christ." The biblical definition of eternal life here is to know. We will spend eternity in an intimate knowledge and closeness with God and Jesus. Wow! And God gifts us with a taste of that in the marital sexual relationship.

Lauren Winner states this well in her book *Real Sex* when she says, "Marital sex is a small patch of experience that gives us our best glimpse of the radical fidelity and intimacy of God and the church" (p. 66). She points out how Paul, in Ephesians 5:32, offers guidelines for how husbands and wives are to relate and then says, "This is a profound mystery—but I am talking about Christ and the church." God gives us the picture of His relationship with the church by showing it to us in Christian marriages. The level of intimate knowing that married partners have—when they are ecstatically, intimately, and erotically bonded during sexual intimacy—is an example of the wonderful, intimate connection we will have with God for eternity. God uses the physical to express the spiritual so that we may know Him.

"Knowing God Guides and Guards our Sexuality." Piper and Taylor do an amazing job of describing this truth in their book. This knowing is the foundation God uses to guard our sexual choices and to guide our sexual lives. When we have that deep, intimate connection with our Father, He not only directs us in how we should live our lives overall, but also in the sexual arena. When we do not retain our knowledge of God, this disorders our sexual lives. "God gave them over in the sinful desires of their hearts to sexual impurity for the degrading of their bodies with one another. They exchanged the truth of God for a lie ... Since they did not think it worthwhile to retain the knowledge of God, He gave them over to a depraved mind, to do what ought not to be done" (Romans 1:24-25, 28; emphasis added). The word knowledge here has the same root, gnosko. When we do not retain or nurture our gnosko—our *knowledge*, our intimate knowing of God—it messes us up sexually.

So let's review. God communicates to us and teaches us who He is through the language of sexuality. His goal is for us to know Him intimately and to have the same intimate knowing within marriage. That knowledge of God can guard and guide our sexual relationships while single or while married. As we progress, we will learn that the Bible includes a wealth of other clear directions on how to live out our sexuality as God intends. This includes when and how we engage in sexuality, who we have sexual contact with and when, how we should view ourselves sexually, how we should talk about sex, and what sexuality in marriage looks like.

Song of Songs

As we mentioned, most of the Scriptures about sex are about what NOT to do. Don't do it with your father's sister, with an animal, with someone you are not married to, or with anyone other than your husband or wife. This is all very clear from the Scriptures. So, when you do have sex, what kind of direction does God give? As mentioned in the Introduction, the Bible is the only world religion scriptural text that devotes an entire book to sensuality and sexuality—Song of Songs. By giving us an entire book about sexuality, God prioritized sex in marriage as beautiful, holy. We need to take note of that. Sensual touch and sensual talk is throughout the Song of Songs. Both the Lover and the Beloved describe each other in sensual, poetic terms. They also use poetic language to describe the delights of the sexual relationship. Note the scriptures below:

Lover: "How beautiful you are and how pleasing, O love, with your delights! Your stature is like that of the palm, and your breasts like clusters of fruit. I said, 'I will climb the palm tree; I will take hold of its fruit.'" The Lover here speaks of climbing the palm tree (her body) to grasp the fruit (her breasts).

Now if you are not and have not been married, you might be saying, "Wait, I am not supposed to read these scriptures, am I?" Valid question. Although a thorough study of Song of Songs would be most appropriate as you prepare for marriage, reading these scriptures to understand God's plan for sexuality is important for all disciples. If you are divorced, it might be difficult to read Song of Songs, as it may remind you that this is not what you had in your marriage. Song of Songs can be both inspiring and depressing, encouraging and scary. If you have any question about whether you should read more of this particular book of the Bible, ask those who are involved in your life and are shepherding you in the Lord. What we can definitely see from this book is that God has intended for married couples to thoroughly enjoy sexuality and the erotic sexual bond with their spouse.

God's Plan of Stewardship of Each Other's Bodies in Marriage

"But a married man is concerned with ... how he can please his wife ... A married woman is concerned about ... how she can please her husband."

1 Corinthians 7:33-34

"The husband should fulfill his marital duty to his wife, and likewise the wife to her husband ... Do not deprive each other except by mutual consent for a time, so that you may devote yourselves to prayer. Then come together again so that Satan will not tempt you because of your lack of self-control."

1 Corinthians 7:3,5

"The wife's body does not belong to her alone but also to her husband. In the same way, the husband's body does not belong to him alone but also to his wife."

1 Corinthians 7:4

You may wonder why we included these scriptures in a book for singles, teens and students. However, many of us have witnessed marriages that have not shown us a godly view of sexuality, both how it should be experienced in marriage and how husbands and wives should treat each other's bodies. Without going into all the detail of how this would look physically, we all need a better understanding of the loving, righteous, thoughtful way that a married couple should interact in their sexual relationship—when they submit their sexuality to the God who created them.

These scriptures in 1 Corinthians 7 have been some of the most specific, helpful, and misunderstood scriptures of the Bible on sex. So let's go over a few important points. God calls spouses to live their sexual lives focused on the pleasure they can bring each other. "A married man is concerned about the affairs of this world—how he can please his wife ... a married woman is concerned about the affairs of this world—how she can please her husband" (1 Corinthians 7:33-34). God calls each husband and wife to consider the other as better than themselves and prioritize the interests of the other (Philippians 2:3-4). If both the husband and wife keep this focus, many of the difficulties in the sexual relationship in marriage will be resolved more quickly.

In a similar way in his letter to the Corinthians, Paul emphasized how someone could be more productive in God's work here on earth if they didn't have to focus on pleasing a spouse (1 Corinthians 7:33-34). Most of us will not choose celibacy. But for those who are married, this scripture makes it clear that a godly husband should be focused on pleasing his wife, and a godly wife should be focused on pleasing her husband.

It is also important to look at who owns whose body according to this scripture. Look at the wording: "The wife does not have authority over her own body but yields it to her husband. In the same way, the husband does not have authority over his own body but yields it to his wife" (1 Corinthians 7:4). Note that for each husband and wife, they yield their own bodies to the other. The word *own* here in the Greek, *idios*, means property. In other words, the wife's body belongs to her, it is her property. As a gift of love, she shares this authority with her husband. It is no longer hers alone, but one to be yielded in love to another. This is a significant point, especially for women. Again, the woman's body, first and foremost, belongs to her. Cliff and Joyce Penner, in their book *The Gift of Sex*, include a chapter titled "By Invitation Only." They discuss how when a woman engages sexually with her husband, she opens up her body. She allows her husband to enter this sacred sanctuary, and this should only be done with her permission. Without that permission, it is a violation. A husband doesn't have the right to force his wife to have sex with him. Nor does a wife have the right to force her husband to engage sexually.

This is very important to understand for women who are not yet married and for young girls. God created your body. You are to be a steward of the body He gave to you. This is also important for men to understand. Remember that no one should ever be allowed to touch anyone's body, especially in any sexual way, without their verbal permission.

There are various ways to understand this idea. Men, if someone just walked into your home and began going into your rooms, randomly opening up your drawers and going through them, you would definitely put a stop to that and consider that a violation. Women, if you have a purse on a table and someone just randomly opens it and starts going through it, you would say, "Hey, what are you doing?" We understand that there are physical boundaries that would be inappropriate to cross without asking. How much more so with the physical body? When making choices about your body, it is vital that the choice, first and foremost, is yours to make.

In marriage, God created the husband and wife to be one flesh, to be unified in both body and soul (Genesis 2:24). Within the spiritual family, we are called to be unified (1 Corinthians 1:10). In the spiritual family, if I consider my brothers and sisters as better than myself (Philippians 2:3), I would not try to force anyone to do something they do not want to do (1 Corinthians 8 and Romans 14). How much more should this consideration apply in the area of sexuality.

In a further look at 1 Corinthians 7, Paul points out that the wife and husband have authority over, *excousia*, each other's bodies. What does that mean? It has often been taught that this means spouses don't have the right to deny their husband or wife's request for sex. This passage has been used in a way that has led to spouses becoming angry or making demands. We have found that through our work with couples, this is in opposition to the heart of the Scriptures and to the overall use of authority in the Bible. If a husband yields part of his authority over his body to his wife, how is she supposed to use that authority? If the wife yields part of her authority over her body to her husband, how is he supposed to use that authority? Jesus taught that the disciples were not to lord it over others the way the Pharisees did (Matthew 20:25-26). Instead, a leader is to be a servant. So when we are given shared authority over each other's bodies, we are to use that authority as Jesus taught: as a servant, not making demands or being selfish. Understanding the scripture as it is intended helps clarify what "do not deny one another" means in 1 Corinthians 7. If both the husband and wife are servants, they will neither demand nor deny. They will give, share, love, and serve. And so each person's body is first of all their own. When a couple unites as husband and wife in marriage, each is deciding that while they retain ownership of their body, God is calling them to share that authority with their spouse and to use that authority to serve. What an awesome responsibility God gives us.

In marriage, as in life, we are to use what God has given us for the good of others. This is similar to the idea of stewardship, taught throughout the scriptures, especially in the New Testament. When someone is a steward, they are chosen by God, given authority by God, to care for something that is really His. We understand this when it comes to money. God gives us money, and we are but stewards of that money while in this life. We are to use that money as God sees fit. This is financial stewardship (Matt 25:20-21, 23). There is also a common understanding that when you borrow something, you should return it in as good or better condition than when you received it.

We know that God has called husbands to imitate Jesus and present their wives as radiant (Ephesians 5:27). These are the concepts reflected in 1 Corinthians 7:4. A wife is given her husband's body from God. He owns his body, but God's will is for him to yield power over his body to his wife. In order to be a good steward of that handsome body, she will do her part to present his body back to God in as good or better condition than when it was given to her. The husband, in the same way, is given shared authority from God over his wife's body. She has granted him that. She is the owner of her body, but he has been commissioned to care for it as for his own body (Ephesians 5:28). God gave him a type of stewardship to nurture and care for that beautiful body. As her husband, his goal is to return it to God in beautiful shape. When he seeks firstto please his wife, he is then able to present her as radiant to God.

How Should a Man and Woman View the Other's Body?

Song of Songs is a poetic love song of how much the Lover and Beloved appreciate, and are drawn to, the beauty of the other's body. It can be difficult to put this in the right context when there are such poor examples in society. A typical movie or TV scene shows two men standing together talking. A woman walks by. The men watch her, focused on her buttocks as she walks by. A woman walks by a group of men and someone whistles or makes a cat call. A man walks by a group of women, and the women make comments and watch his buttocks as he walks by. It is in countless movie and TV scenes, and society has accepted it as the norm. However, it is not in God's plan.

"Anyone who looks at a woman lustfully, he has committed adultery with her in his heart" (Matthew 5:28). And yet, we see in Song of Songs that both the Lover and the Beloved talk very specifically about what they like about the other's body. Sam Laing, in Hot and Holy, says it so well: "His [the Lover's] poetic, rhapsodic language expresses his fascination and arousal and gives honor to the entirety of her divinely given beauty without a hint of demeaning vulgarity… The husband asks… his beloved to let him see her 'form'…"

While single, admiring beauty is one thing. Looking at a body sexually is another. Within marriage, the enjoyment of one another's bodies is a good and godly thing. For women, this can be especially important, to make the distinction between the objectification in the world of the female body and the genuine, godly appreciation a husband has of his wife's body. This is such a delicate balance. Women naturally want to feel admired by the men God has given to love them. They naturally want to feel beautiful. But if that beauty is not admired in the context of the whole beauty of the woman, and at the right time in a relationship, it can lead to an unintended confirmation of that message she's been hearing from Satan and the world: that she is just another body and that she, the woman, is not known and valued.

If this is how sexuality is to be lived out in marriage, how do these things apply to someone who is not married? Paul called Timothy to treat the younger women as sisters (1 Timothy 5:2). So young men and old, when you are not yet married, that is a perfect place to begin treating women's bodies with honor. You can admire her beauty, but you only have the right to enjoy a longer look at a woman's body when you are married to her. More about that in chapter nine, *Purity and Holiness.* Young women and old, the Scriptures give a great example of how to compliment a man's body when you are married to him. Until then, you can admire his beauty, treat him as a brother, and wait to make those catcalls to your husband.

CHAPTER 2

FAMILIES AND SEXUALITY

"Yeah, we had a sex talk. My dad basically said, 'So you know how it all works, right, the whole birds and the bees thing? Great.' And that was about it. Both my parents were too embarrassed to talk about sex."

"My mom would tug my brother's hands out when they were down his pants and swat his hands, and say, 'That's dirty down there.'"

"My mom used to say, 'Where did you get those thighs?' and continually tell me not to eat this or that or I'd get fat and men wouldn't be attracted to me."

"I could hear my parents arguing about sex. My dad would beg my mom, and my mom would just ignore him, and then he'd get angry."

"My dad had *Playboy* and *Penthouse* hidden in his closet. We went to church every week, and heard a lot about how Satan tempts us to have sex, and we need to never think about it 'til we were married. So I got this double message."

"My mom never talked about it with me. Ever. The message I got early on was that it was a taboo subject."

"I think my parents thought if they avoided the topic long enough,
    I'd figure it out on my own."

"My dad's only words of advice were, 'Wear a condom.'"

"When I started to develop, my dad would make comments about
    my breasts getting bigger. I felt really uncomfortable. He
    would always make sexual jokes too. My mom would just
    laugh him off."

"My mom used to say, 'All men are pigs.' She had a lot of
    boyfriends. Several of them violated me; they made comments
    or touched me in really awful ways."

"Most of what I learned about sex was from sitcoms. The clear
    message I got was that men want sex and women don't, but
    grudgingly give it to them to keep the relationship."

"I heard at church ... they taught at school ... my friends always
    said ... I once saw ...."

Do any of these words sound familiar? There are many different things that can influence how a person views and experiences sex, and there is no question that what we experience in the area of sexuality during childhood and adolescence is a big part of that influence. You may have grown up in a family where you experienced a simple and open discussion about how babies are made, and your parents made you feel like you could ask questions. You didn't feel shame for some of the things you felt sexually. That is a wonderful thing.

For many, however, the simple lack of talking openly about sex while growing up has created difficulties in how you experience sexuality as a teenager or adult.[1] Experts in the field of sexual development have found that there are a number of negative sexual events that happen during these

---

[1]   Konzen, J. (2013, November). A phenomenological study of experiences of shame about sexuality for married, evangelical Christian women. Poster session presented at the NCFR Annual Conference, San Antonio, TX. Konzen, J. (2014). The EIS model: A mixed methods research study of a multidisciplinary sex therapy treatment. (Doctoral Dissertation). Available from ProQuest Dissertations and Theses database. (UMI No. 11722)

early years that can have an effect on how you come to view sexuality.[2] The messages at the opening of this chapter may have come from parents, from society, from peers, or from church. However, many of us have also gone through a number of different experiences when we were younger that have given us a skewed view of sexuality.

Researchers say we have a sexual self-schema, an internal map of ourselves as a sexual person (more on sexual self-schema in chapter four, *The Development of the Sexual Self*). They say this self-schema is the way someone thinks about sex, how they view themselves when they have sex, what they think when they look at their own body, and how they think about their own genitals. Negative things that happened to us sexually while we were growing up influence the way we think about sex and about ourselves sexually as an adult. These experiences could include:

- A lack of talking openly about sex in your family
- No (or very little) physical or affectionate touch between your parents or with you or your siblings—no hugs, no holding hands, no cuddling
- Responses from your parents (or someone who took care of you) that were harsh or made you feel shame when you were found touching your penis or vagina
- Very little or no open, honest discussion about changes during puberty like breast growth, having a period, "wet dreams," or a changing penis or testicles

Other negative events include:[3]

- Humiliating sexual experiences or violations (being exposed to pornography, crude or sexual comments, molestation by a family member, friend, or stranger, etc.)

---

[2] Balswick, J., & Balswick, J. (2008). Authentic human sexuality. Downers Grove, IL: InterVarsity Press.

[3] Prager, K. (1995). The psychology of intimacy. New York, NY: Guilford Press.

- Inappropriate or violating kinds of touch (to the buttocks, across the breasts, to the vagina, to the penis or testicles as well as unwanted touches to the thighs, face, neck, feet, hands)
- Witnessing, or being made to witness, adult sex (intercourse or masturbation)
- Having harsh and negative comments made about yours or someone else's body (your weight, size, shape, the food you ate or didn't eat)
- Experiencing any form of physical or sexual abuse (including penetrative sex to the mouth, vagina, or anus)
- Having a parent or someone who takes care of you who doesn't believe you or offer support when you tell them about being molested, assaulted, or touched in a way that was scary, unwanted, violating, or sexual

The women in a research study Jennifer did shared a number of experiences that created negative feelings and beliefs about sexuality:

> "Nobody ever gave me the sex talk, nobody ever told me... I just wish somebody was there to say, 'Guys want this from you, and they're gonna do this and they're gonna say that'... It would have been nice, you know."

> "That's how I grew up. That sex is what you do because you're supposed to. It's not anything voluntary. You just submit to it to have kids."

> "My mom said... 'You have sex with everybody that walks in this house,' and my stepmom said 'You will be pregnant by the end of summer.'"

> "I remember doing it and feeling very guilty and a lot of shame, and I would come home and get on my knees and say 'God, I'm really sorry.' With my first husband, I remember us doing

that (intimate touching) a little bit in the beginning; and on our wedding night, we had sex, and I just cried and cried and cried. 'Cause I was like, how can this... I'm supposed to feel so great about it when I felt so bad about it for so long."

"Just the desire to have it [sex] to me was really sinful, really wrong." "I think also my Mom didn't like any kind of physical affection in front of us, so it made me think it was really dirty or wrong. She didn't like my dad kissing anything, touching or anything... her pushing him away, getting frustrated or flustered when he tried. So I would say I kind of grew up thinking, ewww...ewww."

"I had the abuse when I was little, and ... I always had it in my mind that that was my fault because I was a flirt... I remember even feeling then, 'What did I do that made him think that that was OK?'"

"I think growing up, even thinking about sex was wrong...so I couldn't ask questions."

"I grew up thinking that I wasn't supposed to have it or want it. It's all on the guy's part. They have the desire, and we're just there to fulfill that desire."

"[My mom] heard us looking at each other in the garage, looking at each other's vaginas. Obviously, she'd heard us. But she didn't say much about it. We just didn't go there. She just said, 'If you ever want to know anything about your body or about sex, you know you can always ask me.' And I remember thinking, 'I would love to talk about that.'"

"I think, had it been… not so condemned and not so ashamed, but more understood and taught, I think there wouldn't have been the shame and the guilt and the tears and the fear."

"At some point, she handed me this book called *You Take the High Road*, but we really didn't talk about it."

"I was probably on my period for a whole year before I told her. I just kind of hid it because we didn't have that kind of open communication."

"He was kind of talking to me and kind of following me, and it started feeling a little weird; and he followed me and grabbed me and kissed me, and I like pushed him away and ran. But I would never tell [my parents] 'cause we didn't talk about that stuff. I was sure I had done something wrong. If he would do that, then I must have done something wrong."

"Dad had been very hands on; I mean, we played. He picked me up and threw me around. I sat on his lap. When I was younger. But as I matured, it was very much hands off. Since he didn't want to be inappropriate. I get that to some degree. I didn't have the closeness with my dad anymore. And I really thought there was something wrong with me."

"I think the lack of communication communicated very clearly it wasn't something you could bring up."

"You didn't want to look attractive to anybody. That was sinful. You could cause a brother to lust after you."

Demeaning comments, discomfort with talking about sex, guilt, shame, negative parental sexual relationships, sexual molestation—each of these things skews the development of a healthy view of sex. Though the words above are from women, the reality is that young men also experience negative sexual events growing up. When men talk about their own experiences, they also share about the lack of communication about sex in their families. They talk about the shame or embarrassment they experienced if they were found masturbating and looking at pornography. They mention being handed a book to read about sex with no conversation about it, or hearing their parents argue about sex. Negative comments about the body for boys usually are about their body size, their musculature or lack of muscles, and the size of their penis. Though the number of women who experience molestation and sexual abuse is significantly higher than the number of men, men also share that they had other boys and girls or older men or women violate them. This could have taken the form of demands for oral or anal sex, being forced to engage in unwanted sexual touch with others, or being touched in violating, unwelcome ways. For both men and women, these unwanted sexual traumas might have left memories of feeling pleasure or dark fantasies of re-enacting the event, bringing up another level of shame.

Think about the development of your own sexual self-schema. If you are a teenager, here are some questions to ask yourself:

- How comfortable is it in your family to talk about sex?
- Do you feel like you can ask your parents questions?
- Has anyone ever made negative comments about your body?
- Has anyone made sexually suggestive comments that made you uncomfortable?
- Have you witnessed sex?
- Have you been or are you still exposed to pornography?
- Have you engaged in pornography?
- What fears or reservations have been created by the sexual lives of your parents and those responsible for you?
- Have you been violated by someone?
- Have you ever been touched in any way that felt uncomfortable to you?

- Has anyone kept touching you when you did not wish it?
- If something negative happened to you sexually, did you have someone you could talk with about it? Do you now?
- If you have questions about sex, do you feel like you have someone you can ask?
- Do you feel like there are a bunch of rules about what you're supposed to do regarding sex but not much open discussion or explanation?
- Have you ever had a discussion about self-touch or masturbation with someone you trust?
- Have you ever had someone say something embarrassing or shaming regarding when you touch yourself?
- Are you sick and tired of hearing another talk about purity?
- Have you wondered about whether you are gay, lesbian, transgender, or bisexual and haven't felt like you could talk about it?

If you are a young adult or older single, here are some questions for you to consider:

- In your upbringing, was sexuality a taboo subject in your family, or was it spoken about in ways that felt demeaning, crude, or invasive?
- Did you experience molestation or rape?
- Did you hear negative comments about your body, especially during puberty, or were negative comments made about other people's bodies?
- What was your family's level of comfort discussing the physical and sexual changes during puberty, if they discussed them at all?
- Did your family respond negatively when, as a child, you began to explore sexual sensations and feelings (i.e., genital touching of self or others)?
- Were there rules in your family or in the spiritual environment you were raised in that were never explained, such as whether you should dance, wear certain clothes, go on dates, listen to certain music?

- Were you exposed as a child or adolescent to exploitative sexuality, violating sexual comments, or pornography, etc.?
- Do you have memories of sexual interactions or violations that you felt (or feel) guilty about the pleasure you experienced?
- Did you, and do you, feel like you could talk honestly with someone about attractions you felt to the same sex?
- Did you engage in sexual encounters and you now have regrets?
- Were you ever shamed by someone about how you performed sexually?
- Have you had conversations when you've spoken about your sexual past or sexual sins, and the way the conversation went was difficult for you in some way?

Understanding and talking about your beliefs, feelings, and experiences about sex can definitely be a first step to shedding some light on your challenges that relate to sexuality. Bringing understanding and compassion into this potentially explosive, sensitive area can help broaden the picture of what it is to experience sexuality as God intended.

For some of you, just reading the chapter above might bring up some painful feelings. In the midst of exploring how these negative sexual events may have influenced you, remember God's compassion toward you and any pain you may have experienced. Consider the compilation of scriptures below that expresses God's heart in regards to any scary, painful, or challenging experiences we have in our lives. These are His promises and this is how He cares. As Piper and Taylor have said: "To those for whom sexual experience has resulted in unholy pain, Christ says: 'I understand well your experience. I hear the cry of the needy, afflicted, and broken. Come to me. I am your refuge. I am safe. I will remake what is broken. I will give you reason to trust, and then to love. I will remake your joy'" (Psalm 10, 147; Jeremiah 33; Amos 9).

We have included some exercises below that could be a starting point in opening up with someone you are close to about some of your experiences.

EXERCISES

About the Exercises in This Book

Consider talking with someone about reading this book along with you. You can read certain portions and then discuss it together. This can be a very supportive way of working through your experiences and your beliefs. There are a number of exercises in this book that can help with this. They can be done on your own, with a journal, or in a conversation with someone you trust. Adapt them in any way that is helpful.

The first exercise includes some questions to help you explore sexual events you experienced as you were growing up and how they may be influencing your views and beliefs about sexuality. We would recommend you share with a trusted friend that you are going to be doing this. If you find you begin to experience high distress as you think or write, or if you have any traumatic flashbacks, make sure to take a break and breathe. Then consider if you should get some help from that friend or seek professional support to work through what you are experiencing.

Sexual Background Exercise 1:
Questions to Ponder and Journal

- Did you have a time with a parent or a caregiver when they openly explained about how babies were made and how sex worked (The Talk)?
- When you were going through puberty, was there openness in your family to discuss some of the physiological changes happening to your body? Did you feel able to ask questions?
- Was there much affection in your family (between your parents/caregivers, toward you, among other family members)?
- During childhood, when you began exploring sexual sensations, or touched your genitals, or explored yours or other children's bodies,

did you experience any responses from your parents or caregivers that were negative or that left you feeling shame or confusion?

- When you had sexual questions, did you have anyone you could go to and ask?
- If you have had questions about homosexuality, or if you have experienced attraction to the same sex, did you feel you could talk about it and ask? Or if you did talk about it, how did it go? Have you had confusion or doubt about what you have felt, what others might feel, and what the Scriptures teach?
- Are there scriptures about sexuality that you have questions about and/ or what are questions you have about what the Scriptures teach about any specific area of sexuality?
- Did you receive any negative comments about your body (not just sexually, but overall), or did you get negative messages about your body or about the body overall from any other sources?
- Did you experience any sexually unwelcome or violating experiences (touches, comments, interactions, pornographic material, genital contact, penetration, molestation, rape)?
- Have you experienced any sexual interactions that left you feeling shame? When you think about the words shame and sex, have you had any experiences that associate feelings of shame or embarrassment with sex?

Journal: It may be helpful to take some time to journal your answers to these questions. After answering, explore and write about how you think these experiences may have influenced the way you interact around sexuality as a single, teen, or adult.

Sexual Background Exercise 2:
Mutual Sharing with a Trusted Friend

It is important to have this conversation in a safe atmosphere. It would be beneficial to have a mutual discussion, where both of you share, guided by the questions above in a place where you can be uninterrupted, where there are no time restrictions and plenty of privacy. Also, pray before and after you talk together. Invite God into this tender, sensitive time, remembering that "the eyes of the Lord range throughout the earth to strengthen ("to show Himself strong") those whose hearts are fully committed to him" (2 Chronicles 16:9). Let God bring strength to both of you as you enter this time of sharing.

Trusted Friend: When your friend shares their answers, experiences, and thoughts, listen and merely reflect what they share with you. This would not be the time to interpret or fix or explain your thoughts or view. Simply give your friend a compassionate, listening ear. When it is your chance to share, share openly and genuinely. Give your heart. "Open wide your hearts also" (2 Corinthians 6:11). This can be a conversation that can create a deeper connection in your friendship and that can draw you both closer to God. If emotions or tears are expressed, it can be hard to know how to respond. Sometimes people just want someone to be there for them and listen, or sometimes they need a hug. Ask your friend what they need.

CHAPTER 3

THE NEED FOR TOUCH
AND CONNECTION

One of the topics people are not sure how to address is what we do with touch or our need for touch when we are not married. Those who are single share with us that they hunger to be held; they hunger to feel the arms of someone around them. People have shared that they love going to the hairdresser to get their hair washed because that is one of the rare occasions they receive positive, comforting touch. Sometimes, concern that touching could become sexual with someone of the same sex keeps people from reaching out for or giving caring, comforting touch to their sister or brother. Dating or engaged couples wonder how much they should engage in touch. Parents wonder if they should change how they touch their children as they grow older. These questions can make people feel confused about what kind of touch they should engage in.

Teens and campus students can sometimes receive negative messages from others when they engage in large group lounging or when they are hanging out in mixed-gender groups. Single adults share about the lack of touch in their lives; in some cities, to address this need, professional cuddlers offer non-sexual cuddling sessions. This need even comes up in the medical field. In hospitals, volunteers, or baby cuddlers, give their time to hold and cuddle sick and premature babies. We need touch.

So how do we get it when our culture, either our society or our church culture, may seem not to provide, or allow for, an acceptable way to do it? How can we engage in it joyfully without crossing into touch that becomes sexual? Group lounging can be refreshing and comforting, but it can also lead someone into sexual feelings and thoughts that can make maintaining purity difficult. Many are longing for touch but obviously do not want to have to purchase it, get ill, or fall into sexual sin in order to receive it. So talk about your personal experience and feelings with someone of wisdom that you trust. Share what you do and don't engage in and pray for your own wisdom. "Your Father knows what you need before you ask Him" (Matthew 6:8). God already knows what your needs are. Talk to Him. "The pagans run after all these things, and your heavenly Father knows that you need them" (Matthew 6:32). Take your needs to Him. Rather than running after getting those needs met through your own efforts, lean on Him. He knows and He cares. Talk to Him and talk to someone who is older, wiser, and compassionate.

Let's explore further the importance and experience of touch.

The Importance of Touch

Touch was important to Jesus. Though He could heal people without touching them (Matt 8:13; Matt 12:13), He still touched the leper (Matt 8:3), touched Peter's mother-in-law (Matt 8:15), held a girl's hand as He brought her back from the dead (Matt 9:25), touched an attacker as He healed his ear (Luke 22:51), and touched a deaf man's tongue and the inside of his ears (Mark 7:33). He touched or even wanted to touch His enemies, desiring to gather and enfold under His wings those who wanted to stone Him (Luke 22:51, Matt 23:37). He held children, took them *in His arms*, and put His hands on them (Mark 9:36, 10:16).

Jesus was so personal about His touch. When a woman was healed by touching His garment in the midst of a large, moving crowd, He stopped everything to find out who had touched Him (Luke 8:45). He held the smelly, dirty feet of His disciples, washing them with water (John 13:5). He firmly grasped Peter's hand after he got scared walking on water (Matt 14:31). And how amazing it must have been for the boy who had been possessed by a shrieking, violent demon to look up and see the hand of Jesus reaching out to lift him up (Mark 9:27). What a claim the Scriptures make—that all who touched Jesus were healed (Matthew 14:36). Yes, His touch brought physical healing, but He also touched people just to reassure them, hold them, help them be safe, and serve them. There is no doubt that these kinds of touches brought healing in other ways. As followers of Jesus, our touch can reflect His—showing kindness, reassurance, and compassion. A simple hug can make someone feel safe and show them their worth. A warm touch to someone in distress can bring about emotional healing. Giving in this way provides the opportunity for someone to receive touch from others in a way that makes them feel loved, safe, healed, and believed in.

Touch within the Family

In the field of mental health, I (Jennifer) have come to appreciate the work of Virginia Satir, who revealed a number of different things about touch. Satir was a great believer in the power of touch and its potential for congruent, genuine communication.[1] She found that both men and women experience *skin hunger*, and she believed that one of the greatest things we can lack in our culture is intimacy expressed through the sharing of warm feelings and warm touch. This is particularly true for men, who often have only four acceptable kinds of touching available to them in today's world: the superficial handshake, the firm but quick bro hug or knuckle punch, aggressive contact sports, and the sexual encounter.

Satir believed men's skin was just as hungry as women's and that when people don't touch or when they have different unspoken taboos

---

[1]   Satir, V., Stachowiak, J., & Taschman, H. (1994). Helping Families to Change. New Jersey: Aronson

against touch, their lives can become very sterile. In therapy, she coached married couples to reclaim the enjoyment of warm touch, and she coached parents on how to interact with their children. Satir taught that families can become in danger of cheating themselves if they do not engage in affection; families will often unconsciously develop overly rigid rules to keep touch from becoming sexual. Sometimes, if a child's need for touch is shamed and sent underground, the rest of their senses can end up going underground as well. It is important to understand that healthy, affectionate touch is a vital part of healthy development.

Mothers and fathers, because of their own experiences and fears about sexual abuse and molestation, can become so worried about touching their child inappropriately that they find themselves withholding touch from their children. There can be a lot of confusion about physical affection and touch between family members. The ability to experience safe affection can become impeded by the fear that physical affection would appear sexual in nature, which can also make any discussion of sexuality and any affection taboo. It can be challenging to find that line between enjoying healthy, affectionate touch and respecting the boundaries of others.

This confusion for physical family members about the line between affectionate and sexual touch can influence the same confusion between spiritual family members, brothers and sisters in the fellowship of believers. There can be a lot of questions about the meaning of hugs, about when touch could be considered sexual or lead to something sexual (frontal hugs when a female's breasts touch a male's chest), what kind of touch is appropriate with a same-sex attracted individual, how people touch during prayer, whether to put a hand on a knee, and so many other wonderings. A hilarious video that pokes fun at this conundrum was spotlighted at a Christian conference in 2017 in St. Louis. We highly recommend watching this in order to have a lighthearted way to open up the conversation on our comfort levels with various types of affection: (Search: "Reach2016 - Hugging" on YouTube).

Touch and Mental, Physical, and Relational Health

In the mental and physical health fields today, there is a considerable amount of research on touch. Warm touch, such as massages, cuddling, hugging, and hand-holding, is connected to increased oxytocin (i.e., the cuddle hormone that decreases stress and increases feelings of contentment), decreased blood pressure and heart rate, improved cardiovascular circulation, and reduced stress hormone levels in the cortisol activation response to stress (the chemical responses in the body related to anxiety and stress).[2] When babies are held, they cry less; when deep coma patients receive warm touch, they have improved heart rates.[3] Warm and loving touch lowers anxiety and improves health. Healthy touch improves work and athletic performance. Touch has a therapeutic effect on ADHD, diabetes, migraines, asthma, and immune functioning. And yes, waitresses who lightly and briefly touch the hands or shoulders of customers get higher tips.[4] People who experience lower levels of affectionate touch have lower self-esteem.[5] In fact, those who go without physical touch often experience a kind of skin hunger—that strong desire and need for human physical connection. We definitely need touch.

For couples, touch can cause arousal, but it also soothes and comforts.[6] People often feel like touch is an expression of warmth and support, especially in the midst of conflict.[7] In fact, when a couple gives

[2]   Holt-Lunstad, J., Birmingham, W., & Light, K. (2008). Influence of "warm touch" support enhancement intervention among married couples on ambulatory blood pressure, oxytocin, alpha amylase, and cortisol.

[3]   Field, T. (2003). Touch. Cambridge, MA: MIT Press.

[4]   Crusco, A., & Wetzel, C. (1984) The Midas touch: The effects of interpersonal touch on restaurant tipping. Personal Social Psychology Bulletin, 4(10), 512-51.

[5]   Fletcher, G. & Overall, N. (2010). Intimate Relationships. In Baumeister, R. & Finkel E. (Eds.), Advanced Social Psychology. New York: Oxford University Press.

[6]   Johnson, S., & Zuccarini, D. (2009). Integrating sex and attachment in emotionally focused couple therapy. Journal of Marital and Family Therapy, 36(4), 431-445. doi:10.1111/j.1752- 0606.2009.00155.x.

[7]   Smith, J., Vogel, D., Madon, S., & Edwards, S. (2011). The power of touch: Nonverbal communication within married dyads. The Counseling Psychologist, 39(5), 764-787. doi:10.1177/0011000010385849.

and receives appropriate affectionate touch, their intimate connection deepens.[8] On the other hand, couples who are less affectionate often express that they are less satisfied in their relationship.[9] This can be especially important for those close to marriage. For some Christian couples, waiting until their wedding day for that first kiss is meaningful and noble. But this could also mean they do not engage in what might be considered appropriate, enjoyable, healthy touch that can be an integral part of the natural progression of intimacy leading to marriage. The question for these couples might then be, how do we guard ourselves from sexual immorality and yet feel the freedom to enjoy normal, appropriate affection? (More extensive detail on this in chapter twelve, *Save Yourself.*) It is important to know, even for the unmarried among us, that ongoing affectionate touch in marriage makes married couples feel happier with their sex life, and it makes them feel more comfortable talking about their sexual relationship.[10] Couples who cuddle, kiss, and caress more have higher satisfaction in their marriage and in their sexual relationship. In fact, husbands or wives who say they are uncomfortable with affectionate touch often experience additional roadblocks in their relationship.[11]

So, if touch has so many benefits—physically, personally, and relationally—why don't we do it more? How do we go about discussing it and how do we change things so that we can give it to one another? And if it is so helpful, why doesn't everyone enjoy it? You might be someone who really doesn't like to be touched. On the other hand, you might be someone who constantly feels the need for more touch. Both of these

---

[8]   Mosier, W. (2006). Intimacy: The key to a healthy relationship. Annals of The American Psychotherapy Association, 9(1),34-35.

[9]   Fletcher, G. & Overall, N. (2010). Intimate Relationships. In Baumeister, R. & Finkel E. (Eds.), Advanced Social Psychology. New York: Oxford University Press.

[10]   Heiman, J., Long, J., Smith, S., Fisher, W., Sand, M., & Rosen R. (2011). Sexual satisfaction and relationships happiness in midlife and older couples in five countries. Archives of Sexual Behavior, 40, 741-753.

[11]   Punyanunt-Carter, N. (2004). Reported affectionate communication and satisfaction in marital and dating relationship. Psychological Reports, 95, 1154-1160. doi:10.2466/ PR0.95.7.1154-1160

responses, and others, can be related to the fact that many of us have not always experienced touch as a positive thing.

Problematic Touch

Though we need touch, it is not uncommon for people to dislike certain types of touch. This could be tied to a number of different factors: the emotional state you are in at the time; negative experiences you had as a child or teenager involving touch; if you are ill or have chronic pain; or when you are in the midst of conflict. When conflict is high in relationships, whether a romantic relationship or with a family member or friend, warm and reaffirming affection often disappears because someone is angry or they do not feel safe. Some people need touch in conflict and others hate touch when they are upset. Let's take a closer look at your background to see what is affecting you.

Trauma can affect how someone feels about touch. You may have experienced physical or sexual abuse when you were younger, which may have had a strong effect on how you feel about touch now. If you have continued to experience intrusive or violating touch in adult intimate relationships, this can have a powerful influence on how you feel even when someone gives what is considered positive touch, like a hug. I (Jennifer) worked with a woman who had been raped when she was eighteen. One day, as she stood talking in her church fellowship, a man came up from behind her to give her a whole-body hug. She reacted violently, pushing him away. She was distressed by her own reaction; however, it was completely understandable in the context of what she had experienced. This rather intrusive touch was done without warning and without her permission, which for most would be alarming to some level; but for someone with a background in sexual trauma, this can be devastating. Working through trauma can be an important step in gaining or regaining a positive experience of touch. However, even for those who have not experienced a trauma such as rape or molestation, unexpected touch can bring up a number of different challenging reactions for many different reasons.

You may remember disliking touch as a child. Perhaps you quickly shrugged off hugs and avoided or quickly ended any affection initiated by others. Or you may have had relatives or friends who demanded hugs and kisses. As an adult, you may have experienced an increase in the enjoyment of touch in romantic relationships, though this may have faded with time or when the excitement of a new relationship waned. For those of you with kids, the enjoyment of giving and receiving touch may have increased strongly after you had children. Parents experience pleasure in holding their infant, cuddling with their toddler, and receiving hugs from their child. Other parents with small children report feeling *touched out*, like everyone wants a part of them. Some, however, perhaps due to never enjoying touch, find it hard to hold or touch their children, even though they have the desire to be more affectionate. These different experiences can lead to guilt, frustration, and disconnection.

There are a number of other issues that affect how we experience touch. The need for touch can change according to someone's emotional state. During emotional distress, you might dislike certain kinds of touch or not want any touch at all. Some of you want to be held when you are upset or sad. Others of you do not want to be touched while feeling that vulnerable, though you still might want someone to stay with you as a supportive presence. You might feel OK about a light hand on the shoulder or the knee at the appropriate time that says, "I am here." More than that might be difficult. And the quandary over this need can be especially problematic for men in cultures that do not foster, or may even disparage, the importance of touch for boys and men. Culture and societal norms can have a significant influence on how much men receive warm touch.

Physical pain also influences how people desire touch or how they feel about receiving touch. You might have a family member with a chronic illness or chronic pain who pulls away from touch. It can be helpful to understand the physiological reasons behind their reaction. This is especially true for those with neuropathy associated with lupus, as well as for those with diabetes, kidney disorders, surgeries and chemotherapy, chronic pain, or infections. When people battle these kinds of chronic illnesses, touch can literally be painful. When they pull away, you might feel rejected even though you keep telling yourself it isn't personal and you are trying to be understanding and compassionate.

For some of you, you don't feel there is a lack of touch in your life. On the contrary, you feel like there is too much. Some people express how they feel smothered or irritated when people are affectionate with them, so they begin avoiding touch. Others dislike constantly being touched, but they either do not voice how they feel or only address it when they become angry or irritated. If you have a low tolerance for touch, this may have caused conflict with those you are close to and can be hard to talk about.

For any of you who experience these responses to touch in your relationships, it can be very healing to start discussing the feelings you have when someone touches you or how you feel when it seems like you're touch deprived. If any of these passages describe you, spend some time talking with someone you trust about this chapter. It is important to have a conversation that is free from judgment. Touch can be a very touchy subject (pun intended).

Self-Examination

In our relationship, Jennifer is the one who enjoys touch more. I (Tim) have always been somewhat annoyed by those who show what I feel is too much affection in public, especially when they make out when other people are around. I've been known to shout, "Get a room." I have had to learn the importance and value of touch, both in our marriage and with our children. Jennifer and I have had to talk about touch and affection in our relationship and in our family any number of times. We ourselves are a work in progress in this area.

If you are anything like us, you may be asking yourself, where do I start? Below we have included some steps to help you along the way.

EXERCISE

Communication Exercise: Touch

#1: Examine your own thoughts with some of the questions below. When is the last time you talked about your thoughts on touch and affection and what you need in that area? It can be helpful to first identify how you feel about touch.

- Are you naturally affectionate?
- Do you struggle with wanting more touch?
- Are you feeling touch deprived and experiencing skin hunger?
- Have you been married before or in close physical relationships before, and you are missing the body contact?
- Do you tend to be someone who gives too much touch—touch that could make people feel smothered?
- Do you dread touch?
- Do you avoid someone who is approaching you to give a hug?
- Do you get irritated when someone is touching you too much?
- Do you feel confused about when you should and should not touch someone?
- Are you someone who longs for more affection but you are single and you feel uncomfortable saying something?

#2: Share with someone you trust what you learned from this chapter. What hit you as you were reading?

#3: Consider some questions or frustrations you feel about touch—the lack of it, the dislike of it, the need for it, or your beliefs about it.

#4: Hug each other. The apostle Paul ends several of his letters with a similar phrase: "Greet one another with a holy kiss" (1 Corinthians 16:20, 2 Corinthians 13:12, 1 Thessalonians 5:26). Peter did as well: "Greet one another with a kiss of love" (2 Peter 5:14).

We need touch. Talk about it.

The Development
Of Sexuality

CHAPTER 4

THE DEVELOPMENT OF
THE SEXUAL SELF

How do people develop their beliefs and feelings about sex? This is the question behind the study of how people develop sexually. Learning how your sexuality developed during childhood and adolescence can lead to greater self-compassion and understanding towards others. This knowledge can empower parents to share more confidently with their children about sex. It can empower teens or singles with the self-awareness that parents wish they had when they were younger. When sex is discussed positively in the family, this prepares the ground for how children feel about sex as they continue to grow. If as a child you had negative experiences around sexual topics, this may have created confusion about sex or it may have even lead to addictive behaviors during childhood and adolescence. It can also create challenges in how you live out your sexuality as an adult.

Let's lay some important groundwork to self-understanding, by covering some of the challenges that may occur during childhood and adolescence that impact our view of ourselves sexually, even into adulthood. As you read, think about your upbringing and how it has impacted how you view and live out your sexuality.

Note to parents: Chapter fifteen on "how to talk to your child about sex" will give parents enriching ways to raise their children with a biblical grace-full view of sexuality, even if that wasn't their own personal experience.

Stages of Sexual Development

Knowing the importance of this, let's shore up our understanding of the common stages of sexual development. Though ages are suggested, they are merely approximations and not hard boundaries. Your experience may be different. So let's drop any sense of judgement or shame, and approach this topic with curiosity. We will explore what are considered normal sexual activities and exploration during these various stages of sexual development. By the end of this discussion, you'll have a much better idea how you or someone you love came to view sexuality.

Prenatal. Human sexuality begins at conception. During the prenatal stage of sexual development, Male sperm, with an X or Y chromosome, joins the female ovum which contains two X chromosomes. For most, the combination results in either an XY (male) or XX (female) child. However, in some rare cases chromosomes may instead combine to create a child with XXY, XYY, or XO (only one X). Also, differences in hormonal production can lead to a child who has mixed genitals (both testes and ovaries, or both vagina and penis). As you can imagine, each of these rare cases come with their own set of challenges in sexual development and whether someone prceives themselves or is perceived by others as either male or female.

Infancy. As infants, it is not uncommon for babies to be born with enlarged genitalia due to the rush of hormones at birth. As they grow, infants respond to touch from caregivers. Babies may also derive pleasure or comfort in touching or exploring their own genitals. Lack of loving, appropriate touch during this time of development can lead to challenges throughout life physically, mentally, and psychologically.

Preschool. During the preschool years, children typically begin to engage in mutual touch, wrestling, touching, and kissing. Between the ages of two and five, children are openly curious about their bodies and others' bodies. They can be fascinated by bodily function and sexual genitalia and may engage in individual and mutual exploration. Rather than shaming children for their sexual curiosity, giving affirmation and positive communication along with calm teaching can aid in healthy sexual development at this stage. Suffering from verbal, physical, or sexual abuse or being exposed to exploitative, dehumanizing sexuality at this time can have a devastating impact on the development of healthy sexuality. During these preschool years, children may or may not engage in play that falls into line with our usual expectations of gender. Pushing rigid expectations according to gender (boys play with guns; girls play with dolls) can influence the development of sexuality and intimacy skills.

School-age. Between the ages of seven and twelve (Freud called this the latency phase), interest in sexuality may appear to go underground, though in actuality it is still very active. Children continue to seek out gendered play in order to understand masculine and feminine interactions. For instance, girls may chase boys around the playground (or vice versa). Children also start to become socially aware of what is considered appropriate touch. Sexual play may naturally decline as children begin to keep their questions, interests, and experiences more hidden due to increased social awareness or hearing that something might be inappropriate. By kindergarten, the average girl knows the term sexy, though use of the term increases with age. At this age, boys and girls can begin to be aware of their body shape and may become concerned about weight or what seems "jiggly" or extra flesh. Exposure to mass media's version of sexuality increases exponentially as children approach the middle school years.[1] However, in today's culture of early exposure to electronics and the Internet, a vast majority of children have been exposed to sexually explicit material at this earlier stage.

Preadolescence. In much of today's society, during preadolescence, age nine to twelve, young boys and girls could be very much aware of sexuality due to online exposure. The pressure to be "sexy" and "like a stud," even if children haven't identified these terms as such, has begun. Body image concerns dramatically increase during this stage. With increased curiosity and the beginning surge of hormones, exploration of the genitals becomes common, especially for young boys as they approach puberty. It is also not uncommon for young girls to experience greater amounts of self-touch at this stage. This is also a stage of growing autonomy (the drive to independence) and may show less affection or even be embarrassed to be seen with their parent or caregiver. Masculine and feminine identities can become more strongly identified, or children can wonder (or have felt at an earlier stage) if they are different than a typical boy or girl (see chapter seven, *Sexual Identity Development*). By being warm and approachable, parents can play a key role in the healthy development of sexuality during these years.

Adolescence. The years between eleven and seventeen are a time of enormous change due to the hormonal shifts during puberty. Typically, testosterone surges for boys and estrogen surges for girls. Puberty changes occur about two years earlier for girls than boys. During this time, ovaries and testes mature while secondary sexual characteristics develop such as pubic, facial, underarm, and body hair, enlargement of the testicles and breasts, and changes in the voice. For girls, puberty culminates in menstruation, which typically occurs between twelve and thirteen but can occur as early as eight or nine and as late as sixteen or seventeen (though there are some outside of those ranges). Hormones can cause any number of emotional challenges during these years, and there can be

---

[1] Kilbourne, J., & Levin, D. (2009). Sexy so soon. Ballantine Books.

high anxiety around sexually and socially charged subjects such as bras, dating, deodorant, shampoos, hairstyles, and clothing. Sexual risk-taking can increase dramatically and may involve the use of substances. Engaging in masturbation and viewing pornography increases tremendously for both girls and boys, though societal expectations of boys and sexuality tend to lead to assumptions that girls do not engage in masturbation and pornography.

Research has shown that active involvement in church does influence when teenagers become involved in a sexual relationship.[2] However, the majority of teenagers, including many of those involved in church, engage in sex with partners during these years, primarily through either intercourse, anal sex, or oral sex. Also, intimacy skills can either develop during these years or that development might become stuck or delayed due to varying factors.

What Is Normal Sexual Development?

Normal is a challenging word. What exactly is normal? And just because something is "normal," is it welcome? It may be helpful to understand what are some of the common sexual experiences during childhood. Worried parents call us and ask about things their young children are doing, worried whether it is normal. If a young boy has engaged in touching and being touched by other young boys, is that normal? If a young child has exposed her breasts to someone, is she normal? If preschool age cousins touch each other, is that normal? If he watches other children while they pee, if they reach out and touch dad's penis and mom's pubic hair, if siblings touch each other while taking a bath or shower, if they touch and play with their penis or vagina, if they put objects into their vagina, are these things normal?

The word "normal" has a lot of different meanings, but it is true that

---

[2]   Atkins, D., Baucom, D., & Jacobson, N. (2001). Understanding infidelity: Correlates in a national random sample. Journal of Family Psychology, 15(4), 735-749.

most young children engage in some or all of these behaviors. Three- and four-year-olds love to watch each other as they use the toilet. Parents sometimes find their children playing doctor (looking at and touching each other's genitals). So yes, during early childhood, these are common sexual exploring behaviors. However, just because something is normal or typical does not mean it is welcome. Also, if there is an age discrepancy (i.e., a three-year-old with another three-year-old versus a three-year-old with an older elementary or middle school age child), this may be cause for more concern.

It is common for young children to be curious and to explore sexually with other similar aged children, but this touch may make them uncomfortable or be unwelcome. Often, they do not always know how to express this. We do mention in chapter fifteen on *The Talk* that parents should take this as an opportunity to teach their child to be assertive about what they do and do not want to do, especially in terms of the body. And obviously, if any kind of touch is done coercively or by an older child who is using the younger for sexual exploration, there should be immediate intervention, support, and teaching.

Could these behaviors indicate that a child has been exposed to sexual molestation? They could, and we will cover that below. However, it is important to know that kids do explore and touch, and wonder and question. This is all a normal part of development. Think back to your own development. You likely have your own stories of childhood sexual play. This is important for parents to remember as they respond to these exploring behaviors. What wasn't helpful to you as a child? What would have been helpful?

As children move into the school-age years, they may no longer engage in sexual exploration or openly talk about it when they do because they have become socially aware that doing those things is no longer appropriate. You might think, "My child doesn't think about these kinds of things. They never talk about it." However, their lack of asking questions or doing these behaviors does not mean they are not thinking about them. In fact, grade school children are still thinking and wondering a lot about sex, their bodies, and other people's bodies. And they are hearing things—usually from classmates and their classmates' older siblings.

It is important not to interpret your child's silence to mean they are "too innocent" to have sexual thoughts, feelings, and questions. They have often just learned to conceal their interest and hide their behaviors. One of the most common things that older kids tell us is that they wish their parent had found a way to open up the communication to make it okay to talk about these things. Even at an early age, kids have questions and feelings and are not sure how to start the conversation.

During those same years and into middle childhood—those years from preschool to early and middle elementary school, before a child is on the threshold of puberty—there are some ways that kids explore sexuality that may be cause for concern. They may put their mouths on each other's genitals, they may use sexually seductive language or engage in what looks like sexually seductive behavior. They may imitate sexual thrusting or even attempt intercourse. They might continue to put objects into their anus or vagina. All of these behaviors are important to talk openly about. There are times when these behaviors are reflective of exposure to sexually explicit material, such as pornography. They can also be indicators of sexual abuse. However, it is important to emphasize that these behaviors are not automatically a sign of abuse. They are an opportunity to have some needed conversations. Though these things may not be the result of abuse, they are definitely opportunities to teach boundaries, to teach about sex, to teach about how our bodies are made by God, and to teach appropriate touch. If it becomes known that these behaviors are a reflection that a child has had some form of sexually violating experience, openly talking can be the first step to healing. It is also important to realize that if you were abused as a child, this may be a chance for you to examine if your experience of abuse affects how you see things with your children.

Research on the Development of the Sexual Self-Schema

The sexual self-schema. Each of us has a sexual self-concept, or self-schema. This is an internalized belief or view you have of yourself as a sexual person, including your personal attractiveness, self-worth, gender, sexual performance, attractions, desire, emotions, attractiveness, and body image.[3] Our views and beliefs about ourselves are built throughout life and are reinforced through family, friendship, work, community, and romantic relationships. Childhood and adolescence is also a time when we begin to progressively learn skills on how to relate to others on deeper, more intimate levels.

Difficulties in relating with others during these years of development does influence the ability to gain intimacy skills for future relationships. Therefore, parents should actively promote good relationship skills with their children during these years.[4]

There are a number of different things that can affect the development of intimacy skills and the view someone has of themselves sexually as an adult:[5]

- whether sex was viewed and talked about positively at home
- the level of emotional security within the family (love, affection, acceptance, encouragement, open expression of emotion)
- positive physical touch during childhood and adolescence (affection from parents to children, affection between siblings and other family members)
- if parents had a negative response if a child touched their genitals or explored their body
- cultural views of the meaning of sexuality (sex is for having

---

[3] Andersen, B., & Cyranowski, J. (1994). Women's sexual self-schema. Journal of Personality and Social Psychology, 67, 1079-1100.

[4] Prager, K. (1995). The psychology of intimacy. New York, NY: Guilford Press.

[5] Balswick, J., & Balswick, J. (2008). Authentic human sexuality. Downers Grove, IL: Inter- Varsity Press

children, all men want sex, wanting sex is wrong, how the church views sex)

- positive or negative comments during puberty
- quality of meaningful same and opposite sex friendships during childhood and adolescence
- rigid gender, occupational, and sexual roles and expectations (what toys a girl or boy should play with, what types of chores males and females are expected to do including mom and dad, what type of careers they are expected to pursue or jobs they should have)

The timing of when an adolescent goes through puberty influences how they view sexuality.[6] Boys who are late to reach puberty are sometimes less confident about themselves sexually and more self-conscious about their lack of muscular physique or perceived lack of manliness. Girls who go through puberty earlier may be self-consciousness about their breast size, which sometimes causes them to cover up their bodies.

As mentioned, adults (i.e., parents, teachers, therapists) can sometimes have negative reactions to what might be considered normal sexual behavior in children.[7] They might not take something their child has done seriously or they might overreact and become intensely emotional, angry, worried, or controlling. Conversely, they may fail to react seriously enough, dismissing their child's experience or concern.

It is important to remember that a parent's positive approach to sexuality has an important influence on how an individual views themself sexually.[8] Teenagers who see their parent as both open and adaptive are

---

[6] Rutter, M. (1971). Normal psychosexual development. Journal of Child Psychology and Psychiatry, 11, 259-283.

[7] Heiman, M., Leiblum, S., Esquiline, S., & Pallitto, L. (1998). A comparative survey of beliefs about "normal" childhood sexual behaviors. Child Abuse & Neglect, 22, 289-304.

[8] Murry, V., Brody, G., McNair, L., Luo, Z., Gibbons, F., Gerrard, M., & Wills, T. (2005). Parental involvement promotes rural African American youths' self-pride and sexual self-concepts. Journal of Marriage and Family, 67, 627-642.

more likely to disclose sexual issues to their parents.[9] There are a number of different areas of the parent/child relationship that can create a greater openness about these subjects.[10] These include:

- emotional closeness in the family
- genuine openness on the parent's part
- a good quantity of quality communication
- nurturing interactions
- warm affectionate touch
- overall positive family context

Shame. Sexuality can be a significant source of shame. This is especially true during the teen years when feelings of insecurity can be so strong. Feelings of shame can be connected with negative body image, sexual urges, sexual abuse, or memories of feeling sexual arousal or pleasure when they were sexually abused. Teenagers can also feel a lot of worry about whether they are functioning normally sexually, but they may be too ashamed to ask. The culture and society an adolescent has grown up in, including in their religious upbringing, also influences feelings of shame.

Cultural experiences of shame and sexuality. Research has shown how every culture has different views about sex. Let's look at some examples that have been reported in research in order to have a better understanding of how your own cultural background could be influencing how you view sex and how you view yourself as a sexual person.

Latina women can have a great amount of discomfort talking about sex, using sexual terms (i.e., penis, vagina), or seeking out medical care

---

9   Papini, D., Farmer, F., Clark, S., & Snell. W. (1988). An evaluation of adolescent patterns of sexual self-disclosure to parents and friends. Journal of Adolescent Research, 3, 387-401.

10   Halverson, L. (1994). The effects of childhood touch on the touch patterns of married couples and how they touch their children. Dissertation Abstracts International Section A, 54(7-A), 2466.

for sexual health.[11] Asian women have shared how they avoid sexual topics, including talking to their mothers about menstruation.[12] In fact, in the Japanese language, words for genitals use written characters that imply shame, bashfulness, and the need for negative secrets. Researchers in Hong Kong found that 10 percent of the college students who did a personality test did not answer the questions related to sex, showing a common reluctance to discuss and disclose sexual practices, behaviors, and attitudes.[13] Sex in China is often a taboo subject. Chinese parents are resistant to discussing sex at home, and teachers are uncomfortable teaching about sex beyond mere biology.[14] When sex is discussed, it is in the context of bodily organs and biomedical concerns. American Black women have shared about sexual stereotypes that are byproducts of slavery, when Black women were seen as promiscuous or sexually aggressive,[15] and how these affect how they are perceived by sexual partners. Bangladeshi women in the slums experience shame, stigma, and abandonment if they are found to have a white vaginal discharge, which is believed to come from sexually transmitted diseases.[16]

---

[11] Cashman, R., Eng, E., Siman, F., & Rhodes, S. (2011). Exploring the sexual health priorities and needs of immigrant Latinas in the southeastern United States: A community-based participatory research approach. AIDS Education and Prevention, 23(3), 236-248.

[12] Sandberg, S. (2011). Embodying intimacy: Premarital romantic relationships, sexuality, and contraceptive use among young women in contemporary Tokyo. Dissertation Abstracts International: Section A. Humanities and Social Sciences, 71(7-A), 2524.

[13] Cheung, F. (1985). Cross-cultural considerations for the translation and adaptation of the Chinese Minnesota Multiphasic Personality Inventory in Hong Kong. In J. N. Butcher & C. D. Spielberger (Eds.), Advances in personality assessment (Vol. 4, pp. 131-158). Mahwah, NJ: Lawrence Erlbaum Associates.

[14] Cheung, F., & So, H. (2005). Review of Chinese sex attitudes & applicability of sex therapy for Chinese couples with sexual dysfunction. Journal of Sex Research, 42, 93-101.

[15] Stewart, M. (2010). Perceptions of sexuality by African American patients on hemodialysis. Available from ProQuest Dissertations and Theses database. (UMI No. 3397819)

[16] Rashid, S. (2007). Durbolota (weakness), Chinta Rog (worry illness), and poverty: Explanations of white discharge among married adolescent women in an urban slum in Dhaka, Bangladesh. Medical Anthropology Quarterly, 21, 108-132.

These are just a few examples to illustrate how different cultures exhibit levels of discomfort and shame in the area of sexuality. Sharing your own experiences with someone could expand your understanding of how culture has influenced your views about sex.

Religious experiences of shame and sexuality. The term sex guilt describes a mixture of feeling one should be punished for violating religious standards of proper sexual conduct and that sexual sin cannot be forgiven.[17] Churches can sometimes teach about sexuality in a way that makes it seem like all sex is shameful. For women especially, this can lead to problems, such as body image issues when they do have sex both before and during marriage,[18],[19],[20] as well as feeling like experiencing pleasure in the marital sexual relationship is wrong. When Christian women marry, they can often feel dirty when they do have sex, even within the covenant of marriage. For women who believe they should wait until marriage to have sex, if they do engage in sex before marriage, they often share that they feel despoiled, demeaned, and desecrated.

According to the Scriptures, when we sin, we are called to have godly sorrow and a right kind of guilt that leads to repentance (2 Corinthians 7:11). This kind of repentance leads to times of refreshing (Acts 3:19). However, for some, it can be much more difficult to feel forgiven of sexual sin. Overall, Christian women experience more sexual guilt and shame than Christian men,[21] which may possibly be tied to how women

---

17   Mosher, D., & Cross, H. (1971). Sex guilt and premarital sexual experiences of college students. Journal of Consulting and Clinical Psychology, 36, 27-32.

18   Daniluk, J., & Browne, N. (2008). Traditional religious doctrine and women's sexuality. Women & Therapy, 31(1), 129-142.

19   Reissing, R., Laliberte, G., & Davis, H. (2005). Young women's sexual adjustment: The role of sexual self-schema, sexual self-efficacy, sexual aversion and body attitudes. The Canadian Journal of Human Sexuality, 14, 3-4. Retrieved from http://www.sieccan.org/index.html

20   Wagner, J., & Rehfuss, M. (2008). Self-injury, sexual self-concept, and a conservative Christian upbringing: An exploratory study of three young women's perspectives. Journal of Mental Health Counseling, 30(2), 173-188. Retrieved from http://www.amhca.org/news/ journal.aspx

21   Alvey, M. (2008). College students' psychosexual health: Late adolescent sexual

in general express more feelings of shame about sex and about their bodies in general. This could also be a result of how some religious mothers use shame, guilt, and the fear of disappointing, dishonoring, and letting down the family to keep their daughters from having sex.[22] Women can also receive a greater number of negative messages from their religious community about women and sexuality.

Religious single men also express feeling shame about sexual choices. They will often avoid discussing problems with masturbation and pornography because they feel shame but do not feel there is a place to speak about their struggles within the church community.[23]

Conclusion

After reading this chapter, we encourage you, as we have before, to think through and write down the parts of what has been shared resound with you. What are your experiences, and how do you think they have shaped how you view sex and how you view yourself as a sexual person? Use the questions below to guide you. Share your answers with someone you trust. It may then be incredibly healing to go back and look once again at how God views sexuality so that you can now have a renewed experience about how to view sexuality and how God wants you to view yourself when you think about your sexuality.

God can bring healing, both when we have been sinned against and when we have sinned. Also, though we may remember any number of wrong sexual choices, God remembers us according to His love. "God made him who had no sin to be sin for us, so that in him we might

---

history, religiosity, and shame. Dissertation Abstracts International: Section B. Sciences andEngineering, 69(4-B), 2651.

22   Baier, M. (2008). A qualitative study of the sexual values held by Southern Baptist mothers and how they communicate these to their adolescent daughters (Doctoral dissertation). Available from ProQuest Dissertations and Theses database. (UMI No. 3108681)

23   Kwee, A., & Hoover, D. (2008). Theologically-informed education about masturbation: A male sexual health perspective. Journal of Psychology and Theology, 36(4), 258-269. Retrieved from http://journals.biola.edu/jpt

become the righteousness of God" (2 Corinthians 5:21). When we follow Jesus, we get to be healed by the Great Healer and we get to become the righteousness of God. How cool is that!

EXERCISES

Questions to Guide Your Thoughts and Discussions

*Remember to pray before examining these questions. Ask God to guide your time. Have a friend available to support you through examining these things. Take some extra time after answering these to treat yourself well, remembering that you are in God's hands.

1. When you consider the different stages of sexual development, what were some of your experiences at those times?
2. As you read about "normal" sexual exploration, what do you remember as a child and adolescent? Of these experiences, have you ever wondered if any of them were not normal? How have you worked or not worked through that?
3. How do you view yourself as a sexual person? And what do you think has influenced that?
4. What experiences have you had sexually that leave you feeling shame?
5. Do you see any way that your cultural background has influenced your view of sexuality?
6. In what way did your religious upbringing or lack of religious upbringing affect your view of sexuality and your view of yourself as a sexual person?

CHAPTER 5

BODY IMAGE

She said:

> "I walked all the way around the whole school to avoid a group
> of kids that would call me fatso."
> "My parents always talked about my big butt... My mom would
> always say, 'So round, so firm, so fully packed.'"
> "They would say things like, 'If you stood sideways and stuck out
> your tongue, you would look like a zipper.'
> "I had a boyfriend that dedicated the song [to me], 'Fat Bottom
> Girls Make This Rocking World Go Round.'"
> "I didn't ever feel very pretty. Definitely did not feel very pretty."
> "[My dad] put my older sister on a scale in front of all of us, [so] I
> wanted nothing curvy, and any body part that was attractive
> I would try to hide it."
> "My mom, she would just never eat at the table. She'd put all
> the food on the table and then always talk about what she
> shouldn't eat. 'I shouldn't eat this, I shouldn't eat that.' She
> still does that."

He said:

> "*Being a footballer, you idolize your footballers...when we see those players running around and all, that puts, kind of an image in your mind, like 'oh that's what I need to look like', 'that's how I need to be',,, Your body percent of fat needs to be... low... like zero.*"
>
> "*I want to look the best I can, to have that classic male, slim, muscley build.*"
>
> "*I want to be muscular, I want to be seen as like, strong, in everything.*"
>
> "*I just wanna kind of fit in, to mesh but not to stand out all of my friends are very slim I would prefer a muscular six pack but that's not ever going to happen.*"

Why discuss body image in a book on sex? The words above are quotes from women in a study on experiences of shame and sexuality[1] and from men in a research study on body image.[2] Most of the women had associations between feelings of shame about their body and shameful feelings about sex. Each of them spoke about how these early comments about or experiences with their bodies affected how they viewed themselves sexually as an adult. They described how they wanted to cover up their bodies during sex, how difficult it was to be naked in front of their spouse when they got married, and how they felt the need to have the lights low or off when they had sex so that their spouse could not see their body.

Most of the men expressed how health, bodily appearance and masculinity were important to their overall sense of identity. Most men in the study discussed wanting to get 'bigger' or to maintain a body that

---

[1]   Konzen, J. (2013, November). A phenomenological study of experiences of shame about sexuality for married, evangelical Christian women. Poster session presented at the NCFR Annual Conference, San Antonio, TX.

[2]   Coffey, J. (2016). 'I put pressure on myself to keep that body': 'Health'-related body work, masculinities and embodied identity. Social Theory and Health, 14(2).

looked 'big and strong.' Their appearance was associated with how they viewed themselves sexually. The authors of this study noted that for men, appearing fit and healthy was associated with being viewed as sexually attractive.

So what would this have to do with the life of a single professional or a college student or teenager? The reality is that if you do not process a positive body image while you are single, it can influence the sexual choices you make both before and after marriage. Also, if you have already engaged in sex, these challenges may have already occurred, causing worry whether you will have the same experience in your marriage. Lauren Winner, in *Real Sex*, explains the need to address these issues for singles. She shares that the basis of any sexual ethic for Christians must be grounded in how a person interacts with their own and other people's bodies. "God's vision for human sexuality [begins] with God's vision for human bodies" (p. 33). If you believe that your body is good, you will be motivated to care well for that body and honor it. If you view your own body as beautiful and formed by God, you can then see that all bodies are powerful, that we should care for them and be thankful for them, and always treat them as worthy of respect and honor. Sexual choices are best made grounded in a biblical view of the body.

"No one ever hated his own body; on the contrary, he keeps it nourished and warm, and that is how Christ treats the church, because it is his body" (Ephesians 5:29). The purpose of this scripture is to teach God's church how to treat the spiritual body of Christ. He uses the human body to make the point. We can learn from this scripture how we are to view our bodies. Paul obviously upholds the idea of loving your body, not hating it. Whether or not you love your body is shown in how you nurture it, how you nourish it and warm it. How you interact with your body, including sexually, is one more aspect of how you choose to know God and abide in Christ.

The Influence of Body Image on Sexuality

As we've discussed, good body image sets the stage for relationship success and spiritual dignity. A woman who is tempted to engage in pre-marital sexuality has a much better chance of withstanding that pull if she remembers that she is God's creation and that God has a great purpose for the body He created for her. A young man who is tempted to engage sexually will have a much stronger motivation to make a stand for purity if he understands that God created his body to accomplish incredible and honorable things.

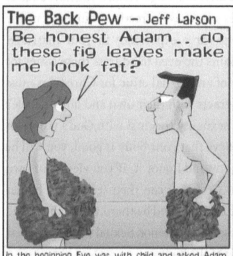

The Back Pew – Jeff Larson

Be honest Adam.. do these fig leaves make me look fat?

In the beginning Eve was with child and asked Adam that age old question... and we all know the correct answer by now. "NO DEAR."

Single and married women often express the desire to feel pretty. But they also share that no one has ever told them they are pretty; they do not perceive themselves as pretty; or their parents, boyfriends, or spouses rarely or never tell them they are pretty. Where women rank themselves against others in beauty and attractiveness (though these concepts are strongly influenced by society and media) can have a significant influence on how they feel about sexuality. Young unmarried women often share that they engage in sex, even when they morally think they should not, because when a man wants to be with them sexually it confirms she must be attractive. Sex then becomes an affirmation of her beauty, that she is good looking enough to be wanted. As we discussed in the previous chapter, figuring out when you started feeling this way can help.

For both men and women, this sense of not being attractive may have started during the pre-teen or teen years. For instance, if you developed sexually early or late, you may still feel unattractive or embarrassed (for instance, women, by the size of their breasts or stomach, and men by the size of their penis or muscles). It is important to work through these issues while single to keep from acting them out in marriage—making you uncomfortable with intimacy or covering up or avoiding being naked with a spouse.

Most of us think of low body image as just a female thing. At least we think women are more obsessed about it! But men have their own set of pressing concerns, including whether they are muscular or thin enough. A survey out of the U.K. found that men also feel the pressure to conform to societal pressures. Three-quarters of the men expressed being unhappy with their body.[3] Surprisingly, men expressed that they would trade a year of their life to achieve their ideal body weight or shape. Eighty percent of the men in this study reported that they had regular conversations with other men about one another's bodies. Sixty percent said that their arms, chests, and stomachs were not muscular enough.

How does this concern come out for a man? When men talk about body image challenges, they express things like feeling small, feeling like they do not have enough muscle tone or enough muscle mass, or being concerned with weight and body fat. Some men only look at their faces in the mirror because they feel that the lack of musculature in the rest of their body makes their body unattractive. Men sometimes wonder if being "skinny" or not having an attractive, muscular physique might be the reason why women are not attracted to them. When men are overweight, they often wonder if their weight is what is keeping women from wanting to date them or be with them.

Men who have high concerns about muscularity are tempted to use supplements and other products, such as steroids, to enhance physique. Men with these concerns are also more likely to start binge drinking and using drugs than their peers. Men do experience eating disorders and can

---

[3]   Franko, D. L. et al. (2015) Internalization as a mediator of the relationship between conformity to masculine norms and body image attitudes and behaviors among young men in Sweden, US, UK, and Australia. Body Image, 15, pp. 54-60.

also be prone to body dysmorphia/muscle dysmorphia (or "bigorexia" in the popular press) with the accompanying distorted view of their own body.

When sharing about the parts of their body they do not like, men have many concerns. They feel insecure about an excessive amount of hair on their body, especially on their backs. They worry about whether their shoulders are broad enough, if their chest is muscular enough (especially if they have unusual nipples or man boobs), whether they have too much or too little facial and chest hair, and if they are carrying too much weight around their middle. They also may worry about other body features (i.e., feet, ears, etc.). Men share how other men made denigrating comments about their body, their weight, or how, when they were younger, boys made fun of the size of their penis. Some men express an overall negative view of their penis due to its perceived smaller size. Others, who are larger, more muscular, and are perceived as more overtly masculine, feel like they are expected to be knowledgeable and proficient sexually.

In general, the concerns with body image for women are usually centered around the stomach, hips, breasts, thighs, legs, and increased fat in the upper back.[4] These concerns for women can lead to avoiding sex or having difficulty reaching orgasm. Men who have compared themselves (or feel others do) to the lean, muscular body image ideal in the media may end up experiencing problems with sexual arousal, pleasure, erectile functioning, and orgasm.[5]

Remember, it is a beautiful and God-given desire to be in a loving relationship with someone of the opposite sex. In fact, many of us start thinking about having this kind of relationship from a young age. (It is not uncommon for women to have their wedding halfway planned years before they are ready to marry). Low body image can short-circuit

---

[4]   Sanchez, D., & Kiefer, A. (2007). Body concerns in and out of the bedroom: Implications for sexual pleasure and problems. Archives of Sexual Behavior, 3, 808–820.

[5]   Basson, R. (2007). Sexual desire/arousal disorders in women. In S. Leiblum (Ed.), Prin- ciples and practice of sex therapy (4th ed., pp. 25-53). New York, NY: Guilford Press.

this desire, causing men and women to avoid romantic or intimate interactions, like dates or playful talk. A husband or wife may also react negatively when their spouse touches their body or they may withdraw emotionally and physically. This can also keep them from being able to relax enough to enjoy sex. All of the individual, relational, and sexual challenges mentioned in this chapter highlight the importance of healing negative body image. This kind of healing work has incredible benefit both for single men and women and for those who enter a married relationship in the future.

So how does someone start that process of healing? One of the first steps to improving body image may be to understand how God views the human body. Most of us are familiar with the scriptures about the body being a temple and that gluttony is a sin. We are often unaware, however, of other scriptures explaining how God views our bodies.

It can also be helpful to reevaluate what influences our view of the human body and how media has a significant impact on those views. Finally, it is vital to learn how to openly discuss body image concerns and explore how these concerns can have a big impact on future and current relationships.

God's View of the Body

"You created my inmost being; you knit me together in my mother's womb."

PSALM 139:13

How does God see the human body? Going back to the creation account, according to the author of Genesis, when God created the world, at the end of each day He declared, "It was good." The day He created Adam and Eve, "male and female He created them" (Genesis 1:27), He said, "It was *very* good" (Genesis 1:31; emphasis added). According to the psalmist, when God knit us in our mother's womb, He did a wonderful work. "I praise you because I am fearfully and wonderfully made" (Psalm 139:14). The Hebrew word, fearfully, or *yare*, means *afright*, to cause awe and astonishment. The Geneva Study Bible states it well. "Considering your wonderful work in forming me, I cannot but praise you and fear your mighty power." When we look at the pinnacle of God's creation, the forming of the male and female body, it should produce reverence and awe when we see the awesome majesty of God as portrayed in our body. We look at majestic mountains and at the vast and powerful ocean and we praise the amazing power of the Almighty God. Yet do we do the same when we look at the human body?

When you look at another person's body or when you look in the mirror at your own, do you focus on the appearance or are you amazed by the Creator? For most of us, it is probably the former. Just as the above research shows, as a society we tend to focus on weight, fat, and muscles rather than on the intricacy of God's handiwork. The apostle Paul speaks a bit about the body. He calls our body a temple (1 Corinthians 6:19). Many have said that people need to stop doing certain things with their body because they need to treat their body as a temple of the Holy Spirit (1 Corinthians 6:20). However, we often fail to say, "Wow, my body IS a temple." That one shift in thinking can completely change how someone approaches his or her body. Not "I should be treating my body as a temple of the Spirit" but "My body IS a temple of the Holy Spirit."

So how are we supposed to view the body? What does the Bible teach about health, eating, and fitness? We know we are supposed to be filled with awe when we contemplate God's creation of the human body, but where does self-control of the flesh fit in? The Scriptures shed some light on these questions. We are to honor God with how we use the body (1 Corinthians 6:20). We should not be gluttons or riotous eaters (Proverbs 23:2, 20). We are called to be wise and self-controlled in how much we eat and the type of food we eat (Proverbs 25:16). When we do eat and drink, or do anything else for that matter, we should do it in a way that glorifies God (1 Corinthians 10:31).

Jesus grew in both wisdom and stature—mature, bodily strength

(Luke 2:52), and the wife of noble character worked vigorously and had strong arms (Proverbs 31:17). We are to love God with all of our strength (Mark 12:30) and to offer our bodies as living sacrifices to God (Romans 12:1). When we fear the Lord and shun evil, there are health benefits (Proverbs 3:7-8). The apostle John even prayed for Gaius' health (3 John 1:2). We need to control our body in a way that is holy and honorable (1 Thessalonians 4:4) and are called to subdue our bodily passions, i.e., sexual immorality (1 Corinthians 9:27, 1 Corinthians 6:13-18) in order to receive our reward in heaven. We should use our body in such a way as to help others get there as well (Philippians 1:20-22).

Our society has continually changing trends in physical health, fitness, weight loss, and diet fads. Some trends focus on nutrition, health, and overcoming illness. Many of these trends are more like idolatry of the body and are focused on appearance. Some people completely ignore health and medical findings and live in ways that damage their health or harm their bodies. Whatever our

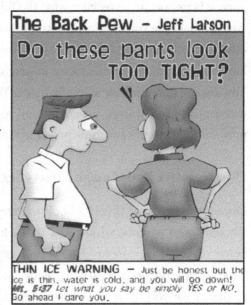

personal view, as a culture, we clearly have a fascination with health, fitness, and the body. Biblically, it is clear that controlling our flesh, using our body for God, and being strong are good and godly things. The danger for many disciples of Jesus, however, is that we can buy into and focus on the worldly view of the body (thinness and muscularity) rather than on feeding the spirit.

Paul warned Timothy of this. He explained that physical training of the body could yield some benefit, but that there was a more lasting, eternal benefit to be found by training in godliness (1 Timothy 4:8). What is important to understand is that the term *physical training* in this scripture refers to refraining from sexual immorality and from eating certain foods. This is not a reference to exercising, such as working out or running. Paul also warned the Colossians that human rules, such as "do not eat" or "do not touch," would have no value in restraining sensual indulgence (Colossians 2:23). These kinds of rules look wise and humble, but are mere human teachings; and, in the end, even research shows that they do not work very well in attaining a healthy body.

In our current culture, with the intense focus on outward appearance, it is important to reclaim what the Bible does say about our bodies. Ask yourself, are you looking at your body as a tool and means to give to others, to promote the gospel of Jesus? Are you aware of how much you have bought into the world's focus on weight, dieting, and the body ideal? You are fearfully and wonderfully made. Your body is amazing and can accomplish great things. When you fail to see your body this way, you may fail to grasp the awesome power of God that is at work in you.

How Negative Body Image Affects Sex

Once again, because this is a book written for Christian singles, teens, students, and parents, why would we include a section on having sex? Some of you have already had sexual experience (either before marriage or in a previous marriage). Body image may have already been a challenge for you in those relationships. Also, for those of you who are hoping to be in a relationship one day, you can do yourself and your future partner an incredible service by working through any issues with body image that you have now so that your sexual relationship can be all God intends. With that in mind, it can help to know ahead of time what some of the challenges might be even in a healthy Christian marriage so that you can go into your future relationship prepared ahead of time for the challenges that could arise.

So, to recap, this research shows that when you have a negative body image or when you have internalized body objectifying comments and images, this can lead you to feeling self-consciousness about your body in intimate relationships and later in marriage. Often, people think that when they are married, all of the insecure feelings they have about their body will just go away. This may be true initially, or early in marriage, but these ingrained views often return with full force later (for some, it happens on the wedding night). Some young married couples, when they have continued to view their bodies negatively, end up experiencing sexual dysfunction (physical discomfort or pain during sex, erectile dysfunction, premature ejaculation, difficulty reaching orgasm). Body image for both men and women has also been connected to lower sexual desire, lack of initiating sex, low sexual frequency, lack of enjoyment, lower sexual satisfaction, and feeling sexually unattractive.[6] When someone has a negative body image, they may have no problem saying no to sex before marriage. Then, during their marriage, they may avoid sex because of their self-consciousness about their body and appearance. For those who are insecure about their bodies, but who wait to have sex until they are married, they might experience a difficult time relaxing enough to enjoy sex when they do get married.

If you have challenges with negative body image, take some time to talk with someone you are close to about how this has affected you to this point. If you have had past sexual relationships, share your experiences. Talk with that person you trust and share some of the concerns you might have about how this could affect your future marital relationship. Then lay all this out before God in prayer.

"He Is Altogether Lovely."

We know that the Scriptures teach that we should not look at someone's body and lust. We understand that if we are not married to them, and we look at them and think sexual thoughts, we are in sin. However, how

---

[6] Cobia, D., Sobansky, R., & Ingram, M. (2004). Female survivors of childhood sexual abuse: Implications for couples' therapists. The Family Journal: Counseling and Therapy for Couples and Families, 12(3), 312-318. doi:10.1177/1066480704264351

should we view other people's bodies even when we are not thinking sexual thoughts?

How do you feel about, think about, and talk about other people's bodies, including your own? This is a loaded question. The world presents a constantly shifting standard of what makes up attractiveness. None of us (even models, actors, and actresses) can measure up. Let's take a look at the one book in the Bible that gives us a clear understanding of how we are to view another person's body. Yes, this is a book full of thoughts and words between two lovers. However, it gives us good insight into how we are to view one another physically. It can also be a good primer for how, when someone is married, they should think about and talk about their spouse's body. And believe us when we say, if you don't have a good perspective now, you will have difficulty having a good perspective when you are married.

Look at how the Lover and Beloved talk about each other in Song of Songs. The Lover says of his Beloved, "You are altogether beautiful, my love, there is no flaw in you" (Song of Songs 4:7). What woman would not like to have someone say this to her, especially someone she is in love with? Look at the words he uses to describe her (4:1-15 and 7:1-9): lovely, delightful, pleasing. And when he speaks of her body, he talks in detail about her eyes, hair, teeth, lips, mouth, temples, neck, breasts, navel, and waist. He even compliments her on her breath and her voice. He tells her she has graceful legs, beautiful sandaled feet, and a lovely face. He says she is like the dawn, as fair as the moon, as bright as the sun, and as majestic as the stars. He sees her as totally unique and special. "My dove, my perfect one, is unique" (6:9).

Consider these words and ask yourself, when you look at women's bodies, do you pay attention to the overall beauty of the body, the lovely feet, the beautiful eyes, or the pretty face? Women, when you look at your own body in the mirror, do you look primarily at your weight, and the trunk of your body, whether it is slim and shapely, or do you also appreciate the other parts of God's creation as it is displayed in your body—the neck, the hair, and the mouth? Do you ever take time to wonder at the marvel of how the parts of your body you cannot see are made? God has included these words in His writings to us to model how we should think and speak about the female body, both ours and others. In fact, women changing how they look at other women is a good place to start how we view the female body.

The Beloved says of her Lover, "Oh how handsome you are, my beloved! Oh, how charming... My beloved is radiant and ruddy, outstanding among ten thousand" (Song of Songs 1:16 and 5:10). What man would not love to have his beloved think about him this way? When she speaks of his body, she in turn describes his head, hair, eyes, cheeks, lips, and arms. She talks about how his body is polished ivory (his protection, 5:14), how his arms are rods of gold (his strength, 5:14), and how his legs are like pillars of marble (again, his strength, beauty, and power, 5:15). When is the last time you focused on how a man uses his body to serve rather than giving undue attention to his buttocks or his muscles, noticing his cheeks, his smile, his expressive eyes, and how he does his hair? How he uses his strength when he helps someone who has to move or when he plays with a child? God has allowed these descriptive words to be included in His inspired Scriptures to call men and women to a higher perspective on how they view and talk about men's bodies.

Men, consider these scriptures and ask yourself, when you look at your own body in the mirror, do you pay attention to all that your body can accomplish and to the amazing creation of God, or do you primarily make a judgment based on muscles and the amount of weight on your body versus someone else's body? Body image is not just a female concern. Men also have a mental representation they create of what they think they should look like and can be concerned with how others view them. Men can often be focused on gaining weight (compared to the typical focus for women on losing weight) and gaining muscle. We are all exposed to the *media* ideal of muscularity (compared to a more balanced view of what muscles are actually supposed to look like), and this can cause men to feel dissatisfied with their bodies.

OK, let's be honest. Sometimes, there are things we do not like about our bodies or that we do not find attractive about someone else's body. So what do we do with that? You *can* be both honest and honoring. If you have extra weight, you can be honest about that, but you can also admire the entire wonder of how God created you. You can be honest with yourself about someone else's body, what is not necessarily attractive to you (without dwelling on it), but then focus on admiring what is beautiful, unique, and wonderful.

One of our favorite examples of this is the relationship between Guy and Cathy Hammond, founders of the Strength in Weakness ministry. Guy is a same-sex attracted man who lived a homosexual lifestyle for over ten years, and who has now been a faithful disciple of Jesus for over three decades. Guy and his wife, Cathy, have been married for over twenty-five years and have four children. Guy openly shares that, even now—though he has not engaged in homosexual acts since he became a Christian—he is still not attracted to the female body. Many who have heard him share this have wondered, "Wow. How does that work between you and your wife?" His response to those bold enough to ask this question out loud is to share in detail how he sees his wife as an amazing rose that is a wonder to behold—a rose that has a long fragile stem and rich, beautiful, soft red petals that release a wonderful scent. What woman would not like to be described in this way?

Cathy also shares very openly when she is asked what it is like for her to know that she does not have the type of body her husband finds sexually attractive. Her response is that she knows, and he knows, that her body will never be able to live up to her husband's sexual fantasy. Still, they regularly compliment each other, telling each other how they find one another attractive. They have made their physical relationship about giving and honoring each other. What an incredible example these two are!

So ask yourselves this: do your thoughts and words reflect a godly appreciation of the human body as found in God's Word? We can all grow and change in this area. When we do, we will honor one another in a way that creates lasting and loving relationships and that fosters confident, godly views of the awe-inspiring creation of the human body. Our purpose in how we use our bodies is to reflect God's image to the world. However, instead of inscribing His image on the world, we can often end up letting the world inscribe its image on us. It is important that we reclaim and redeem the view of the body as it is created in God's image rather than live according to the world's view.

The exercises on the following pages have a number of different purposes. They may expose how media influences your view of your body. They may help you regain a biblical view of your body. They may help you communicate with someone you trust how you feel about your body. These are just a couple of steps that can start you in the direction of reclaiming how fearfully and wonderfully made you are.

* *Cartoons from The Back Pew by Jeff Larson, used by permission.*

EXERCISES

Body Image Exercise 1: Videos in the Media

Watch both of the following videos (or watch them with a friend): A video about women: "Watch Photoshop Transform Your Favorite Celebrities" on BuzzFeed

A video about men: "Before and After Fitness Transformation" on YouTube (Warning: There is bad language used in this video.)

Take some time to talk with someone about what you think about each of these videos.

Body Image Exercise 2: Fearfully and Wonderfully Made

Find a comfortable place in your home. Read all of Psalm 139, and then focus on verse 13. While sitting comfortably, place your hands on different parts of your body, reciting Psalm 139:13, "I am fearfully and wonderfully made." Example: place your hands at your waist or on your upper arm and consider the internal parts of your body below your hands (your tendons, the bone, the veins, your kidneys, stomach, lungs, etc.) and the external parts of your body your hands are directly touching (your waist, thighs, upper arms, shoulders, hips, etc.) and share with God how they are fearfully and wonderfully made.

Speak and pray with God about how intricately and carefully He made each part of your body and how well it works with all the other parts of your body.

Body Image Exercise 3: Mirror

Below is a body image exercise. Read the directions before beginning. Do this according to your comfort level. Each of the sentence prompts are about how you view your body.

While fully clothed, standing facing the mirror, speak out loud about the parts of your body, placing your hand on that part of your body.

- "One part of my body I like is …."
- "Another part of my body I like is …."
- "What I think is attractive about my body is …."
- "One part of my body I am not fond of is …."
- "Something about my body I'm insecure about is …."

* After the exercise, if you are able, meet with someone to talk about what the exercise was like for you. You can also take time to write these in a journal to pray about and talk about further.

CHAPTER 6

SEXUAL ABUSE

"Praise be to the God and Father of our Lord Jesus Christ, the Father of compassion and the God of all comfort who comforts us in all our troubles, so that we can comfort those in any trouble with the comfort we ourselves receive from God."

2 CORINTHIANS 1:3-4

God is a God of hope and comfort who longs to redeem our sexual trauma. If you have a background that includes some type of sexual trauma, you may be looking for hope. Or you may be in relationship with someone who has faced these kinds challenges. It is important to understand sexual abuse and its impact on how we live out our sexuality.

Addressing the challenges that individuals have with a background in sexual trauma, and how it effects their sexuality, deserves an entire book of its own. We have recommendations at the end of this chapter for various books that do that very thing. This chapter is intended to briefly highlight some of the primary challenges that someone can experience in their life as a result of sexual abuse and trauma. We will also include how these experiences can specifically impact intimate relationships. Hopefully, this will be a beginning in helping you find healing and connection if you have experienced sexual trauma or abuse.

We do want to point out that this chapter can be challenging to read for those who have experienced abuse. In order to work through this, you may need to gather around yourself some supportive relationships: a close friend and advisor, a trusted family member, a spiritual mentor, or a counseling professional. Be aware that you could become triggered as you read; be sure to seek the help you need through this time.

It is important to state here that our society can tend to think that women are the primary victims of sexual abuse. The statistics somewhat bear this out. Women do experience sexual abuse at a higher rate than men. The National Sexual Violence Resource Center (NSVRC) says that 1 in 4 women have been sexually abused before the age of eighteen and 1 in 5 women have been raped in their lifetime. In my (Jennifer's) work with women, I would say over half of the women I work with—both professionally and in the ministries I have led—have experienced some form of sexual abuse or molestation. Men, however, are also victims of rape and sexual abuse. NSVRC reports that 1 in 6 men experience sexual abuse before the age of eighteen, and 1 in 33 men have been victims of rape.

Young men might not report abuse for various reasons, including beliefs that "real men" should be able to protect themselves, that others might think they are gay, or that they must have been complicit in some way because their penis was erect during the abuse. Young girls might not report abuse because they fear that they will not be believed, they feel protective of the abuser, or they are afraid of getting in trouble. There can be so many difficult reasons even for an adult male or female to not report a sexual assault. "They might retaliate," "Everyone would hate me if I told," "I might get blamed," "I might lose my job," "I don't trust the police."

For these and many other reasons, if you have been the victim of sexual assault during childhood, adolescence, or adulthood, the difficulty of making a report and the experience you had can continue to have an ongoing effect. Both men and women who've had these traumatic experiences share that they feel like they did something wrong, that there is something wrong with them, and that they are not sure if they are now too damaged to have a quality sexual life with their spouse.

The Effects of Sexual Abuse and Trauma

There can be a number of significant effects on those who have experienced physical and sexual trauma. Survivors express that they feel guilt and shame, experience flashbacks, and have challenges in intimate relationships. Sexual abuse can also cause physical illness, physical trauma and injury to the pelvis, depression, anxiety, fear, helplessness, anger, health problems, gastrointestinal issues, mental health challenges, problems with concentration and attention, hypervigilance, nightmares, eating disorders, self-harm, sexual risk-taking, hypersexuality (or sexual promiscuity), or suicidality.

There can also be lingering self-blame. I have worked with men and women in their fifties and sixties who will share their stories of how they were assaulted many years ago. They often still attach to their story words like:

> "I shouldn't have let him in, gotten in that car, gone to her room."
> "I still feel guilty about feeling that... saying that... doing that... responding in that way."
> "I should have left... should have told... should have known."
> "I could have stopped. I could have said no."

They often tell me they know it wasn't their fault, that they were a child, that they were young and did not know, or that they felt they had no power. But even when they mentally recognize that, they feel they were still somehow at fault.

A woman who was part of my research study shared that when someone did something inappropriate to her as a child, she would later ask herself, "Was it my fault because I was a flirt?" She even answered that question with, "I think I was a flirt at a really young age," but that she thought it was for attention and just wanting to have someone want her. "I always felt like I kinda promoted it (the sexual assault) because I was such a flirt." In a similar response, male survivors have shared, "I responded sexually, so I probably gave some kind of signal that it was something I wanted."

Some men and women experience shame in association with abuse, but they do not have anyone to talk to about it. The lack of a safe place to talk can lead to internalized shame messages. At the time of the abuse, they may have hidden what happened. And they might still desire to hide as an adult. One woman shared how she did not feel she could tell her parents:

"When I was about twelve or thirteen, I remember being in a hotel with our parents, and they let us go down in the video room and play games and stuff. And there was a man, he was a lot older than me. He was kind of talking to me and kind of following me and it started feeling a little weird, so I went and took the stairs up to my parent's room. He followed me and grabbed me and kissed me, and I like pushed him away and ran up the stairs. And I remember going into my hotel room, and just saying, 'I got to go to the bathroom' then going into the bathroom and being like 'huuuh, huuuh,' you know, just breathing and freaking out that that just happened. But I would never tell. 'Cause we didn't talk about that stuff. I was sure I had done something wrong, that he would do that. If he would do that then I must have done something wrong. That was like a sexual thing, with a boy, and so, uh oh, I feel like I would have been the one in trouble. Or I don't know, just like it must have been my fault. I must have done something."

Survivors question their worth or whether they are still damaged in some way. One woman wondered if she was "still a good person" and was she at fault for the sexual abuse she experienced.

"I had an instructor ... he came up behind me, I was bending over a cooler, and he grabbed my hips and rubbed his penis up against me, and I thought it was one of the boys in my class, and I turned around and kinda swatted him and then I realized who it was, and I remember even feeling then, 'What did I do that made him think that that was OK?'"

These internalized messages of fault, guilt, worth, and the desire to hide can affect not only an individual's personal life, such as hiding their body within baggy clothes, it can also affect their close intimate relationships. Though the examples shared here are from a study of women, men share similar feelings—either of low self-worth or that they are damaged or perverted in some way. Recognizing and transforming these thoughts and feelings can be a healing process, especially when that process is directed by God.

The Sexual Effects of Sexual Trauma

Sexual trauma can come in many forms, including:

- inappropriate touch (i.e., an older individual touching the buttocks of a younger child);
- exposure to sexually explicit materials or experiences (pornography, watching or being made to watch individuals engage in sex or masturbation);
- exploitative sexual comments (sexual jokes, comments about the body, or harsh and negative responses to sexual exploration)
- sexual molestation and rape (including penetrative and non-penetrative sexual violations).

Though the percentage of women who experience molestation and sexual abuse is significantly higher, men also share how other boys or older men or women violated them with demands for oral or anal sex, or even forced them to engage in sexual touch and sexual contact with others.

Sexual trauma can result in flashbacks. These might occur at any time of the day and in any circumstance. They can also occur during sexual activity. It may have happened to you in a past sexual relationship. It is possible it could happen when you are married. It is important to know ahead of time what could possibly occur and what to do when it happens. For some people, past physical and sexual trauma can cause physical problems with sex. Some women experience ongoing physical discomfort and pain in the vulva, which can be the result of trauma to the tissues or tightening of the muscles due to anticipation of pain (it is important to note that if someone experiences sexual pain, though it can be a result of sexual molestation, it could rather or also be a symptom of a medical issue that needs to be addressed by a sexual medicine specialist). Married men and women who are abuse survivors may also have little or no interest in having sex and may have problems with arousal, erection, and orgasm.

Sexual trauma can also lead to numbing out during sexual activity. Children and adolescents who were physically abused—including victims of rape, molestation, and sexual assault—often express that they withdrew mentally from themselves and the circumstances while they were being assaulted. This is often described as a way they coped with the sheer terror, fear, betrayal, and physical pain they experienced. As these individuals then become involved in intimate relationships, they might find that they avoid sex, have an out-of-body experience during sex, or have a challenging time enjoying sex. What is healthy and protective as a child can become restrictive as an adult.

So it is understandable why some survivors of sexual abuse experience high anxiety about sex and highly negative feelings about sexuality in general. These responses may include a sense that sex is dirty, guilt or fear in expressing sexual preferences (what hurts and what feels good), suppressed anger that reduces desire, and distressing flashbacks. Others experience the opposite. They may become promiscuous, subconsciously seeking to heal past trauma by entering similar situations, trying to gain a feeling of control instead of feeling powerless. As they approach marriage, it is not uncommon for women who have experienced sexual trauma to feel fear about what sex is going to be like with their soon-to-be spouse. This can be especially challenging if you have had other sexual partners before marriage and things have either not gone well or have been painful. Sexual abuse survivors sometimes share that when they engaged in premarital sex, they did not have traumatic responses at that time, but that these responses began occurring after they are married. It is important to share and seek help if this occurs for you.

Sexual abuse survivors may also have unwanted sexual fantasies or disturbing, random sexual thoughts. When they do engage sexually, they sometimes feel powerless during sex, lack sexual assertiveness, have difficulty communicating about sex, or withdraw emotionally during sex. Sexual abuse can result in conflicted feelings about having sex, such as experiencing a desire for sex and not wanting sex at the same time. Survivors can sometimes feel they have no right to sexual enjoyment and often think they just have to learn to endure sex. For some individuals, these various symptoms show up immediately after a sexual violation, while for others they do not show up until years later.

Crisis of Faith

If this is your story, sexual trauma may have left you doubting God. When you've shared this with other well-meaning individuals, they may have dismissed your feelings, either with platitudes such as "God is with you" and "God works out everything for the good" or with equally insensitive responses that make you feel guilt and shame for doubting or being angry with God. You may wonder, why is this happening now? Young children who have been abused do not always question God. However, as they grow older and they begin to explore their own faith, these questions can be uncovered.

Know that you aren't alone in having these thoughts and doubts and that this isn't an indication that you are unspiritual. It is common for those who have been sexually abused or who have experienced sexual assault as an adult to wonder where God was. "Why would He do this or allow me to experience that?" "Where was God?" "If He is the protector, where was He?" Sexual violations can cause Christians to wonder if they are being punished by God.

Taking the time to explore how you view God can be vital to the process of recovery from physical and sexual abuse. Establishing safe, supportive relationships that you can go to when these questions and doubts arise is also important. For an excellent book on the spiritual journey, see *Grace Calls* by Robin Weidner.

Problematic Touch

We discuss problematic touch in chapter three, *The Need for Touch and Connection*, but want to do a brief review here. If you have experienced physical or sexual abuse during your formative years, this can affect how you feel about being touched as an adult. Also, if you have experienced intrusive or violating touch in adult intimate relationships, this can increase the challenges you experience even in a healthy, godly relationship. When someone with a sexual abuse background gets married, they may need to relearn touch, and how to talk about touch, within the safety of their relationship. Wendy Maltz, author of *The Sexual Healing Journey*, provides a video, *Relearning Touch*, where couples can practice the pen exercise, the hand-clapping exercise, the back-writing exercise, the nesting exercise, and others. These exercises help an individual gain a renewed sense of mastery of their own body and control over distressing automatic reactions to touch and sex. They also allow couples to explore healthy touch and an enjoyable sexual relationship. For those who are approaching marriage or who are already married, these might be an important part of learning that sexuality is safe.

Do know that for those who have experienced sexual violations, unexpected touches, especially unexpected sexual touches, can bring up traumatic memories and feelings. When you get married, you may notice that it is upsetting if your spouse touches you without seeing them coming or if they come from behind to touch you. Simple consideration, such as asking permission to touch, may go a long way toward creating safety. Find a way to talk openly about this as a couple, even when you are dating or engaged, or get someone to sit with you as you discuss this so that touch, including the sensual and sexual touches during marriage, can become something that enhances your relationship.

Staying in Your Body

For those of you who remember withdrawing from your body during the abuse or violation, you may have a difficult time staying in your body during sex, even in a loving, godly, married sexual relationship. If this becomes your experience, trauma therapy or sex therapy may be necessary to learn how to manage the fears and automatic responses that often cause you to disassociate from your body during sex. It is very important to note here that this *diassociation*, the feeling that one is observing their own body, is a common, even normal, response to sexual trauma. It does not mean, "I'm messed up." It could mean that you may need additional professional help to work through this very automatic response. You might find both individual and group therapy to be helpful. The process of healing from sexual trauma can help survivors release themselves from blame, recognize that the perpetrator was the one responsible for the sexual violation, and learn to experience a sexual relationship in marriage without fear.[1]

Many times, memories of sexual abuse can be triggered during sex.

---

[1] Cobia, D., Sobansky, R., & Ingram, M. (2004). Female survivors of childhood sexual abuse: Implications for couples' therapists. The Family Journal: Counseling and Therapy for Couples and Families, 12(3), 312-318. doi:10.1177/1066480704264351

If this happens, it may be tempting for an abuse survivor to ignore the traumatic trigger. They may then "go out of their body," like they did as a helpless child. This can then lead to a physical and emotional distance in the marriage relationship. For some of you, these responses may have already occurred when you engaged sexually before marriage. For others, it may occur when you get married. When I work with individuals who disconnect, or disassociate, from their bodies—either during sex or at other times as well—I begin with helping the individual learn how to stay in their body first while they just talk about sex. This can be the first step to calming the anxiety response. It is also essential for healing that each man and woman feels they have the choice whether to engage sexually. It is especially critical for sexual abuse survivors to feel like they are the ones driving the car—that they have control of their own body and rights over their sexual selves. For further reading on ownership of the body, see chapter one, *What Does the Bible Say About Sex?* and chapter five, *Body Image.*

Professional Treatment

Professional treatment for sexual abuse and trauma can include a number of factors and is dependent on the mode of therapy a counselor or therapist uses. Treatment modalities may be group and individual therapy, trauma-focused CBT (cognitive behavioral therapy), prolonged exposure therapy (PE), EMDR (eye movement desensitization and reprocessing), somatic experience (SE), hypnotherapy, traditional treatments for PTSD (post-traumatic stress disorder), art and music therapy, and equine therapy. Traditional treatments might include stress-reducing techniques, medication, journaling, emotion expression, management, and regulation, desensitization, confronting the perpetrator, trauma narratives, and other forms of reprocessing the trauma.

If counseling isn't readily available, there are many ways you can still work on personal healing, even now before you are married. Reclaiming God's view of sexuality can be an incredibly important part of a sexual abuse survivor's journey. The spiritual journey of redeeming sexuality through biblical counseling is often vital to someone's process. If you decide to pursue therapy for sexual abuse from a spiritual counselor, this might include understanding the effects of sexual abuse, reexamining sexual beliefs, learning how God's intent is that marital sex be enjoyable for the husband and wife (this can be especially important for women), learning how to remain within your body when you are in distress or when you are receiving touch, and finding ways to deal with intrusive images and thoughts.

When you do get married, part of the journey of sexual healing may also include getting help and healing as a couple. For instance, as we mentioned, when someone has experienced sexual trauma, touch—even non-sexual touch from a loving spouse—can be very difficult. If you decide to seek couple or sex therapy to help with these issues, therapy might include a gradual approach to intimate touch that is safe, comforting, and eventually sensually and sexually enjoyable.

Whether or not you seek out a professional, it is not uncommon, even within the strongest and safest of marriages, that a survivor's trauma will occasionally be unexpectedly re-triggered while they are having intimate time with their spouse. Finding ways to communicate about these things and building a new experience of safety in connection to sex can provide additional healing for both the individual and the couple.

If you marry someone who has a background of sexual abuse, you may also benefit from counseling, for you might sometimes feel confused, rejected, abandoned, inadequate, or unattractive. It can be helpful to gain an understanding that "sexual healing is rarely as fast as survivors and intimate partners would wish."[2]

---

[2]   Maltz, W. 2012. The sexual healing journey (3rd ed): p.7. New York: HarperCollins.

Healing After Sexual Abuse

"To those for whom sexual experience has resulted in unholy pain, Christ says: 'I understand well your experience. I hear the cry of the needy, afflicted, and broken. Come to me. I am your refuge. I am safe. I will remake what is broken. I will give you reason to trust, and then to love. I will remake your joy'."

PIPER AND TAYLOR, PSALM 10, 147; JEREMIAH 33; AMOS 9

The process of healing from sexual trauma and abuse can be a winding journey. Individuals do flourish. Couples do connect and have great intimacy. Teenagers do go on to do great things and have healthy intimate relationships. God can bring about great victories. Joy can win. And it does. Be open. Be real. Be vulnerable. Seek support. Talk with a group of understanding people. Have a trusted mentor. Build relationships with safe people. Go to God for comfort, for understanding, and for a new experience of love. In that process of healing, we want to share a few verses to support you in that direction. Sometimes we need to hide. Not from God, not from others, but we need to hide in the shelter of His wings. God calls us to make Him our hiding place. In pain and trouble, there we go.

"You are my hiding place; you will protect me from trouble and surround me with songs of deliverance."

PSALM 32:7

"Whoever dwells in the shelter of the Most High will rest in the shadow of the Almighty."

PSALM 91:1

"Praise be to the Lord, for he showed me the wonders of his love when I was in a city under siege. In my alarm I said, 'I am cut off

86

from your sight!' Yet you heard my cry for mercy when I called to you for help."

PSALM 31:21

"How abundant are the good things that you have stored up ... for those who take refuge in you. In the shelter of your presence you hide them ... in your dwelling you keep them safe ... Praise be to the LORD, for he showed me the wonders of his love when I was in a city under siege."

PSALM 31:19-20

"Because of the LORD's great love we are not consumed, for his compassions never fail. They are new every morning; great is your faithfulness. I say to myself, 'The LORD is my portion; therefore I will wait for him'."

LAMENTATIONS 3:22-23

"One thing I ask of the Lord, this is what I seek; that I may dwell in the house of the Lord all the days of my life, to gaze up on the beauty of the Lord, and to seek him in his sanctuary."

PSALM 27:4

"He will command his angels concerning you to guard you in all your ways; to lift you up in their hands."

PSALM 91:11

"'Because he loves me,' says the LORD, 'I will rescue him; I will protect him, for he acknowledges my name'."

PSALM 91:14

"In my distress I called to the Lord; I cried to my God for help. From his temple he heard my voice; my cry came before him, into his ears. The earth trembled and quaked, and the foundations of the mountains shook; they trembled because he was angry. Smoke rose from his nostrils; consuming fire came from his mouth, burning coals blazed out of it. He parted the heavens and came down; dark clouds were under his feet."

PSALM 18:6-9

"Hide me in the shadow of your wings."

PSALM 17:8

"You are my hiding place."

PSALM 32:7

"Rescue me ... for I hide myself in you."

PSALM 143:9

"This is what the LORD says—he who created you ... he who formed you... 'Do not fear, for I have redeemed you; I have summoned you by name; you are mine. When you pass through the waters, I will be with you; and when you pass through the rivers, they will not sweep over you. When you walk through the fire, you will not be burned; the flames will not set you ablaze. Since you are precious and honored in my sight, and because I love you, I will give people in exchange for you, nations in exchange for your life'."

ISAIAH 43:1-4

Take some time to slowly meditate on these scriptures and allow God to begin the process of healing in you body, in your spirit, and in your soul.

Here are some resources we recommend for those who have experienced sexual abuse or molestation:

For Men and Women:
The Sexual Healing Journey, Wendy Maltz
Relearning Touch, Wendy Maltz Video (found at http://healthy-sex. com/booksdvdsposters/dvds/relearning-touch/)

For Women:
Grace Calls, Robin Weidner Website: robinweidner.com

For Men:
Healing the Wounds of Sexual Addiction, Mark Laaser
Evicting the Perpetrator: A Male Survivor's Guide to Recovery from Childhood Sexual Abuse (2010), Ken Singer
Website: 1in6.org

CHAPTER 7

SEXUAL IDENTITY DEVELOPMENT

This is a topic very much in the forefront of the media. It is also very much on parent's hearts, whether it is in regards to their own child or someone else's. However, it is not just a parental concern. It may be heavy on your heart because it brings up questions about your own sexuality or the sexuality of someone close to you. Whether it's a challenge for you or someone you care about, as the spiritual family of God's church, it's important for all of us to have some compassionate understanding of the development of a gay, lesbian, or bisexual identity. To answer the many questions we receive, let's consider the development of same-sex attraction (SSA). Of course, there are a number of different alternative gender identities and directions of attraction, such as bisexuality and transgender identity. Much of this material we share here will also apply to any number of these gender and attraction concerns.

Often the focus on talking about same-sex attraction is for males and the gay community. But this is also a female issue. As a church family, we need to consider how to have loving, healthy conversations and relationships with sisters who are experiencing same-sex attraction as well.

One of the most common questions about same-sex attraction is how does someone become attracted to the same sex? Some of the most common assumptions is that this is the result of having an overprotective mother and dismissive father, or an uninvolved mother, or ... in whatever imaginable way, it was the parent's fault. Another common explanation is that the individual experienced sexual abuse, especially sexual abuse from a same-gendered person. The reality is, there is very little verified research support for these assumptions. What we know for sure is that there are plenty of SSA individuals who were raised by supportive, involved, balanced, loving parents. Also, though the percentage of same-sex attracted individuals who have been sexually abused is higher than the general population, only a small percentage of those who have experienced sexual abuse become same-sex attracted. Making blanket assumptions like these can actually shut down healthy communication about these very tender issues.

The other primary question people have is whether SSA is genetic or biological. This is reflected in the popular song, "I Was Born This Way." In today's culture, this is a huge question. Is same-sex attraction something someone is born with? The short answer is there is no definitive answer. There are a great number of complex factors that go into sexual formation, and this is true of same-sex attraction. Christian households sometimes have another spin on this question, "Is same-sex attraction natural?" The scripture commonly asked about is Romans 1:26-27:

"Even their women exchanged natural relations for unnatural ones. In the same way, the men also abandoned natural relations with women and were inflamed with lust for one another."

At a plain reading level, the words natural and unnatural seem to indicate that it is not the natural state for someone to engage in sex with someone of the same gender. Let's delve deeper into these difficult questions: *Is someone born this way; what is the process of sexual formation for SSA individuals,* and *how should we respond?* You might be reading this as a same-sex attracted individual. You may be a parent. There may be someone you love expressing these feelings. We hope you find what we include below helpful. If you need more direction beyond understanding the development of same-sex attraction, we would highly suggest the work of Guy and Cathy Hammond, with the Strength and Weakness ministry at strengthinweakness.org.

Born This Way

Can we know for certain where same-sex attraction comes from? The American Psychological Association has this statement:

> "Although much research has examined the possible genetic, hormonal, developmental, social, and cultural influences on sexual orientation, no findings have emerged that permit scientists to conclude that sexual orientation is determined by any particular factor or factors."

A recent review of the research suggests, regarding the origins of sexual orientation:[1]

> "Despite decades of research, the ultimate answer to the question posed in the title of this paper, 'Can anyone tell me why I'm gay?' is a resounding 'Not yet.' ... While there is some evidence to suggest physiological correlates ranging from genetic markers to structure and function of the brain, one can feel quickly overwhelmed by the sheer amount of contradictory findings on all of these fronts, and the news is no better, if not worse, for research concerning the role that familial and environmental factors play in the development of sexual orientation."

Do note that both the APA and the author of the article are gay-affirming organizations. Their conclusions are that there is no scientific support for any claims that same-sex attraction is genetic. Rather, the number of factors can be numerous. These conclusions fit into the overall

---

[1]   North American Journal of Psychology, 12(2), 279-296.

understanding that experts in the field of sexuality have made about all sexual development. All of the factors mentioned in the APA statement could be at play: genetics, hormones, social/physical/emotional development, society (including family structure) and culture. We just don't know how much biology plays a factor in same-sex attraction, and to make strong statements in either direction is unsupported by science.

Sexual Identity Formation

The work of Mark Yarhouse, a researcher and clinician in the field of same-sex attraction, proves helpful. This is somewhat technical. There are a number of different models that explain the development of same-sex attraction. However, what we review of his work below is a well-researched process of sexual identity formation for same-sex attraction (how someone develops SSA) that includes what Yarhouse calls a valuative framework, a consideration of the morals, values, and beliefs in the process of development and choice of lifestyle. According to Yarhouse, sexual identity includes:

- Biological sex (DNA) and sexual genitals (vulva and breasts, penis and scrotum)
- Gender identity (feelings of being a boy or girl or some combination of masculine and feminine)
- Persistence and direction of attraction (the feelings persist and are primarily in a certain direction)
- Behavior and motivation (physical exploration or engagement in sexual activities, or involvement in online activities, etc.)
- The Valuative Framework (beliefs and values in the home and within the religious environment)

Yarhouse divides the process of sexual identity formation into the following five stages. Though these are focused on gay and lesbian identities, they can also be adapted to the development of bisexuality and transgendered identities:

Identity confusion or crisis: A time period, either in grade school or in middle school, when a child feels different from others of the same gender. These feelings are usually accompanied by confusion and keeping these wonderings hidden, often because these feelings seem incompatible with their or others' beliefs.

Identity attribution: The period when someone begins to put meaning (attribution) to their same-sex attractions. The meaning might include a denial of the experiences of SSA (I feel these feelings and attractions but I am not gay or lesbian), or the meaning might be influenced by their values and beliefs (I have these feelings and attractions but they are wrong).

Identity foreclosure vs. identity expansion: This period may include a premature closure (foreclosure) on sexual identity—either a rejection of a gay or lesbian identity or an embracing of that identity —without exploring or examining the beliefs and values that influence these decisions.

Identity reappraisal: When the person reevaluates the initial rejection or acceptance of a gay or lesbian identity.

Identity synthesis: The acceptance and synthesis of the gay or lesbian identity with the overall identity of the person or a disidentification of the gay/lesbian identity. The idea of *disidentification* involves both the acceptance of feeling same-sex attraction alongside a choice, based on an examination of values and beliefs, to not pursue an active gay or lesbian lifestyle. These individuals find that identifying as gay or lesbian is inconsistent with their religious identity.

Let's Put It Together

OK, so what does all this mean? There are a number of different things that affect the development of same-sex attraction as well as bisexual attractions. This includes the family and religious community someone grows up in. It also involves how someone feels about their body, especially the sexual parts of their body, and whether they feel like a boy or girl (and how families respond to various masculine or feminine tendencies). SSA individuals begin to have feelings of attraction toward someone of the same sex, and others may find they are attracted to both sexes. They may begin exploring those feelings physically, or they may experience sexual violations. They may also begin to explore this on the Internet.

As they grow older, they might begin to realize that these feelings go against their beliefs or their family's or church's beliefs. During this time, they may feel confusion, and it may cause a crisis emotionally or psychologically. As they develop, they will place different meaning on these same-sex or bisexual feelings, and they may fluctuate between accepting and rejecting, hiding or speaking about these feelings and experiences. At different points, they may explore these attractions in light of their own growing understanding of God, the Bible, Jesus, and the church.

Now the big question—how do we respond? If you are thinking of someone else, your job is to be there with them as an example of God the Father. If this regards your own journey to figuring out who you are, knowing God and your identity in Christ can also provide light and direction.

How to Respond

Love. Support. Empathy. Hugs. Listening. Having Fun. Hugs. Sharing. Reading. Playing. Hugs. Encouragement. Praise. Listen some more. Hugs. Eat. Laugh. Pray. Hugs.

Carefully look at each of these words. Check how each of them are going for you. And DO NOT withhold your affection. If someone you love shares that they are same-sex or bisexually attracted, listen and hug them. Allow them to talk. Speak about your thoughts with love, patience, and respect. Read the paragraph above (Let's Put It Together) and put yourself in their shoes (if you are not the individual with SSA). Sexual formation is confusing and anxiety producing for everyone at some level, no matter their sexual attractions. There is an incredible amount of angst during the preteen and teen years even without experiencing the confusion of being attracted to those of the same sex.

It is also important to remember that the years of adolescent development and early adulthood can be marked by many questions and doubts about sex, sexual attraction, and sexual identity. It is not uncommon for teens or singles to wonder if experimenting with or having thoughts about sex with someone of the same gender means they are gay or lesbian. However, thoughts or experimentation are not the same as gay and lesbian sexual identification. Give room for open conversations about these wonderings and questions.

We need to look at Jesus. How did He respond to people? When He was healing people, He touched them. And most of the time, He didn't even need to. As we talked about in chapter three, *Need for Touch and Connection*, we see that although He could heal people from afar, He still took their hand, held them, and lifted them up. Be affectionate. Also, have your conversations in private. When Jesus healed the deaf man who could not speak, He took him aside, away from the crowd. Make sure that you have conversations in private and then keep those conversations confidential. If you are dealing with SSA and need to get help and support, make sure those you speak with are a reliable few and that they will keep your confidence. If you are helping others with SSA or bisexuality, make sure you get their permission to tell the specifics of their story to those you turn to for advice. We recommend that you even share with your child or your friend exactly what you are going to ask and make sure they are okay with that. This is vital to create safety in your relationship with them.

Ultimately, Jesus cared deeply. When you see Him at the funeral for the widow who had just lost her son, the Bible says, "His heart went out to her" (Luke 7:13). In the Greek, the term *splagchnizomai* means His guts were moved. Jesus was moved at a visceral, gut level. This is such an incredible example of empathy. His heart was deeply moved. Jesus was respectful, loving, and direct. After challenging her accusers, He told the woman caught in adultery (John 8) that He did not condemn her. And then He told her to "leave your life of sin." We can be both loving and direct. We can speak the truth and we can do it in love.

In John 4, Jesus met the woman at the well and He talked with her. He engaged genuinely, lovingly, and personally with her and then he talked about how she was living with a man who was not her husband. Jesus did not avoid the challenges but he did surround them with love and care. He told the rich young ruler, whom he loved, to sell everything he had (Matthew 19:21). That young man went away sad. Jesus shows us the perfect mixture of grace and truth, of love and challenge, of support and direction. We can give all those things as well. Set your eyes on Him and imitate Jesus.

Remember these scriptures:

"Always be prepared to give an answer to everyone who asks you to give the reason for the hope that you have. But do this with gentleness and respect" (1 Peter 3:15). "Those who oppose him he must gently instruct" (2 Timothy 2:25). "Fathers, do not exasperate your children; instead, bring them up in the training and instruction of the Lord" (Ephesians 6:4). Be gentle. Be respectful. Don't exasperate. Speak the truth and do it like Jesus. Remember that you yourself "were bought at a price" (1 Corinthians 6:20). Keep your eyes on the cross and pray to imitate Jesus.

For Parents: Your Teen Believes It Is Okay for Someone to Be Same-sex Attracted.

In today's world of instant access to information, and with the prominence of societal, political, and religious conversations about SSA, your child is wondering. They are having a conflicting number of thoughts. They have friends who are same-sex attracted, and they are hearing gay affirming words in their school communities. The best thing you can do for your child is to make it safe to have these conversations with you. Draw out what they are thinking. Let them speak their mind. Give weight to their thoughts, their conclusions and their arguments. They are often very good arguments. If as a parent you use platitudes, or those quick "God made Adam and Eve not Adam and Steve" arguments, you will shut the conversation down and fail to engage your child in a way that connects them to God and His Word. Absolutely share your convictions. Just remember to speak the truth in love, and keep the conversation open. Ask them how they feel about what you share. We recommend coming back to this conversation as often as needed without inundating your child in a way that makes them tune you out.

Your Child Is Same-sex Attracted

It is very common for parents to feel devastated when they discover that their child is attracted to the same sex. Parents express that they feel how they do when they have lost someone. They are walking around with a devastating pit in their stomach. They are angry, confused, and scared. This might describe you. And what you are feeling is completely understandable. You may be married to someone who has a different response. "They will be fine." This doesn't mean that your spouse doesn't care and doesn't love our child. Though this may feel dismissive of the grief or fear you experience, we encourage you to remember that every parent deals with this kind of issue in a different way. Remember, you need support. Your spouse and children need support. Your child needs a loving parent, parents who love each other (if you are married), and good friends. Get help. Get support. Talk and get advice and direction before you respond if your first tendency is to attack. If your child says they feel like you are attacking them, listen and get with someone to talk through this. God is big enough. God cares and He mourns with us when we mourn. Parents, be that for one another and always remember to be a messenger of reconciliation (2 Corinthians 5:18), for each other, for your child, for their friends, for your friends, and for all others you know with SSA. For the rest of you reading here, read *Caring Beyond the Margins*, by Guy Hammond, a same-sex attracted individual who supports those experiencing SSA.

Remember that "The Lord gently leads those that have young" (Isaiah 30:11). He is gentle with all of us while calling us to imitate Him.

"Be imitators of God, therefore, as dearly loved children and *live a life of love*, just as Christ love us."

EPHESIANS 5:1, EMPHASIS ADDED

Live a life of love and show the world who God is.

Sexual Feelings
And Practices

CHAPTER 8

SEXUAL ANATOMY 101

"So God created man in His own image, in the image of God He created him; male and female He created them."

GENESIS 1:27

As we went to work on creating this book for singles, teens, students, and parents, we did briefly wonder whether we should include education on anatomy. Well, duh! Why would we wonder about that? Often, we can think that if we talk about sexual anatomy and how sex works, this might lead to someone going and having sex. And hence, in a book for Christians who are not married, our goal is not to promote having sex, right? However, this whole quandary is the crux of the issue.

Within the Christian culture, this misconception that silence promotes purity is deeply rooted, but there is a very destructive plant that grows from that idea. Lack of information, resulting from the idea that talking about sex is taboo, can result in naïve or misinformed choices. If we are not lovingly given this information from those we trust spiritually, our only option it seems is to get it from other less trustworthy sources, such as the Internet. After all, the Internet is a great resource to help us make good and godly decisions for our sexuality (we hope you can hear the sarcasm here).

So let's start reversing this trend. The people who should be the most open and honest about sex should be Christians who believe in the God who created sex. Let's cast away our fear-filled responses and embrace how God created the sexual body. Then, we can approach how God wants us to live out our sexuality with all the joy and confidence He intended us to have.

God created man. And yes, that means that He created the penis. God created woman. And yes, that means that He created the vagina. When you look at our sexual organs in and of themselves, you may wonder just what He was up to. It will be an interesting question to ask Him one day. We do know that God created the human body to enjoy sex. Yes, He did. Anatomically, the greatest number of nerves are found in the genital organs. However, being sexual is much more than just about our sexual organs or just the act of sex.

The brain is involved in sex and is actually called the most important sex organ. The brain receives all the signals and sends out all the instructions involved in sexual activity (including communication to the nerves and all of our senses). The brain regulates all of the chemicals involved in sexual interactions, including inhibiting sexual responses, as well as increasing the blood flow, respiration, and perspiration, and organizing all the emotions and memories associated with sex.

In the last several decades, there has been a growing understanding of exactly how the sexual parts of the body work and what kind of biological processes take place during sex. This chapter is devoted to understanding the physiology of sex. We recommend that both men and women read all the sections, including both male and female sexual physiology. After all, you took the class in middle school, you learned about it in physiology in college, or you looked it up on the World Wide Web. Let's do it here while we marvel at the wonder of God's design.

"God saw all that He had made, and it was very good" (Genesis 1:31). Note: The following section goes into explicit detail on the male and female anatomy. If you are in the process of overcoming sexual addiction, seek counsel from those whom you trust if reading about the details could cause a relapse. You may then want to skip ahead to the section on purity and how to respond to arousal. You also may want to consider having that trusted friend join you in reading this material in order to gain a new understanding of sexuality and to aid you in your pursuit of recovery. Also, if you have a background in sexual abuse, speak with those with whom you are close about whether you should read this together with someone you trust to provide support. If you are a single disciple and reading about male and female anatomy in this kind of detail creates some challenges with your purity, seek counsel about the best way to approach this section.

Imagine sitting with a group of students at a church event. You are getting ready to have a class on purity. Woohoo! You are so excited. Not! You have heard this lesson over and over. Don't do this. Don't do that. Then the speaker gets up and says, "I have a question for all of you. Have you ever watched a movie, or listened to a song, or read or seen or thought something and your vagina started throbbing or your penis became hard?" As the noise in the room and the uncomfortable laughter get loud, you look around and realize that this is the most bizarre class on purity you've ever heard.

And yet, isn't this the place we should be having that discussion? In God's family. Our bodies are built to become sexually aroused. If we are going to talk about pursuing purity, we had better face the fact that our bodily response is a part of that pursuit. So how exactly does arousal work and what do we do with it? The first thing we are going to look at is what exactly is happening when you think that thought. What are all the bodily parts involved in sexual arousal?

Male Sexual Anatomy

Male external genitals are primarily made up of the scrotum, the shaft, and the head of the penis. Within the shaft are the three erectile columns (think of column shaped sponges) with veins running through them providing blood to the penis. These columns are called the corpus cavernosum (two columns) and the corpus spongiosum (one column). The corpus spongiosum is the tube of erectile tissue that surrounds and protects the urethra. Picture a mechanical pencil where the outer column (the corpus spongiosum) surrounds the thin pencil lead (the urethra).

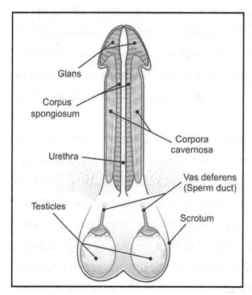

The head of the penis includes the most sensitive part of the penis, the glans, and the coronal ridge, which circles the head of the penis at the base of the glans (in the diagram, you can see the coronal ridge beneath the glans). Along the underside of the glans, perpendicular to and crossing the coronal ridge, is a ridge of tissue called the frenulum (this is not shown in the diagram).

An elastic skin structure in the circumcised penis surrounds the entire shaft. This elastic structure includes the foreskin in the uncircumcised penis (circumcision is the removal of the foreskin usually done shortly after birth). The tissue at the base of the penis between the testicles and the anus is the perineum (not shown).

The scrotum is a suspended sack of skin that holds the testicles, where sperm is produced. After leaving the testicles, sperm travels through the pelvic cavity by way of the vas deferens (two thin tubes, one from each testicle). Each vas deferens narrows and then passes through the ejaculatory duct. The vas deferens then joins with the urethra as it passes through the prostate. Semen, the milky fluid that is ejaculated during orgasm, is produced by the prostate gland and the seminal vesicles and is combined with sperm as it passes through the prostate (not shown). The sperm and semen mixture is then sent to the penis via the urethra for ejaculation. The penile and scrotal structures are anchored, supported, and innervated by various muscles, ligaments, and nerves within the pelvic floor. Blood brings food to these tissues, the bones and muscles hold everything up and make things move correctly, and the nerves allow you to feel different sensations.

Female Sexual Anatomy

The vulva. We tend to call the female genitalia in the pelvis the vagina. However, the correct term for the entire area is vulva. The vagina is actually the tube that extends from the opening found in the vulva to the internal structure of the cervix and uterus. The female vulva surrounds the entrance to the vagina, and consists of the vestibule (the vaginal entrance), the minor and major labia (the lips or labium majus and minus), the clitoris, the mons pubis, which is the fatty tissue usually covered in pubic hair that

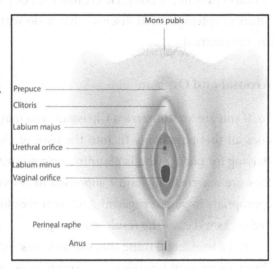

protects the clitoris, and the anterior perineum (perineal raphe), which includes the tissue between the vagina and the anus.

Within the vestibule, above and below the vagina, are two sets of glands, the Bartholin's and Skene's glands (not shown). The Bartholin's glands release lubrication for the vestibule, and lubrication is also released within the vaginal walls. The tissues surrounding these glands are one of the common sites for genital and sexual pain. Most nerve sensation is felt only in the outer third of the vagina (the part closer to the entrance). The clitoris is made up of the head (the glans), the shaft (shown but not labeled), and the crura (the legs or crus clitoris). The crura, or legs, extend around the vagina underneath the labia. Many blood vessels carry blood to this area when the tissue is stimulated. Female erectile tissue, much like the erectile tissue in the penile shaft, surrounds the clitoris including under the labia. When stimulated, these tissues fill with blood as the penis does, causing arousal sensations.

An important note about the nerves to the genitals: Male and female genitals have the greatest number of nerves in the human body. The tongue and fingers also have a great number of nerve endings, but still have less than half the number of nerves as the genitals. God created the sexual organs of the body. He created the body to enjoy sexuality and, in future chapters, we will discuss what to do with that creation when you are not married.

Arousal and Orgasm

So, if you are an unmarried Christian, you may still be wondering, how does all this physiology fit into the plan of God? For someone who is striving for purity, who is planning on refraining from having sex until they are married, how am I supposed to respond to arousal? Is it ever appropriate to pursue orgasm? And what should I do if I have an unsolicited orgasm (i.e., as the result of a dream)?

It is a wonderful thing that the Bible has such a clear answer for this. "Young women of Jerusalem, I charge you: do not stir up or awaken love until the appropriate time" (Song of Songs 8:4). There is a whole chapter in this book dedicated to *Purity and Holiness* (see chapter nine) and another about waiting until marriage, *Save Yourself* (see chapter twelve). However, at this time we want to specifically address what to do with arousal that happens when you're not married.

The first thing we recommend is to realize that arousal is initially a purely physiological response. The throbbing and tingling that is caused by blood flow to the vulva and the erection that is a result of the blood flow to and engorgement of the penis, are automatic physiological responses to sexual stimulation. There are many times when you are not consciously doing anything to cause these sensations. No one is touching you. You are not touching yourself. You are not purposefully looking at sexual photos or videos, or listening to provocative music, or watching a sexual scene in a movie. However, a thought quickly crosses your mind or a brief picture comes in your head. You are watching TV and a Victoria's Secret ad comes on. Or someone kisses someone in a movie. And boom, your vagina throbs and your penis becomes erect. Penile and vaginal engorgement is initially controlled by the lower spine. What that means is that instantaneous flow of blood to the genitals is prompted by the mechanisms within the lower spine, much like a knee jerk reaction. When you are visiting the doctor, he might use a rubber mallet at your knee to assess the automatic reflex in your knee. That is almost exactly how penile erection and vulvar arousal works. It is an automatic reflex to a stimulus. Your thinking brain is not yet involved. If you have done nothing to purposefully cause the response, the initial response is completely involuntary. You can voluntarily choose to cause it to happen by touching the penis or vulva or looking at a pornographic image. You can also voluntarily choose to continue looking at that flash of a Victoria's Secret commercial or dwelling on that romantic/sexual scene, and that's when the thinking brain gets involved.

Why is all this important? God created us with that automatic, knee jerk response. This is so important to understand. Why? God built that response into our body so that when we do purposefully plan to become sexual in marriage, our body will get us ready for the enjoyable act. Physiological arousal, blood flow, vaginal lubrication; they are all a part of the incredible plan God put together to make sex pleasurable and meaningful. Often what happens when a single Christian becomes aware of arousal, arousal they did not intentionally cause, they can feel a certain measure of guilt or confusion. Obviously, if someone awakens sexual love, or purposefully stimulates their body or mind with a touch, a video, or a romance novel, this enters into the area of choice; whether to maintain purity or pursue impurity.

When that *knee jerk* response happens, we can choose to be amazed by God's creation rather than be filled with shame and guilt. We tell people when they experience natural, unintended arousal, to say to themselves, "Wow! My vagina is awesome" or "Look how well my penis works" and "Didn't God do an amazing job creating my body?!" The initial physiological response is a God-given biological wonder. What we do with it from there is what can be guided by our beliefs and love for God. We can then say, "Wow, isn't my vagina/my penis wonderful? Now I'm going to call a friend, sing a song, go on a walk, say a prayer." Our choice on how to respond to arousal is where we put our values about sexuality into practice in order to honor God. But in order for that honoring to happen, we sometimes first need to give credit to the Creator.

So when we become spontaneously aroused, we can choose not to pursue orgasm. We can decide that we are leaving that for a time when we are married when it can be enjoyed with the man or woman God created for us.

What about when that orgasm happens in the middle of the night when we are sleeping? For men, this might include a *wet dream* when the penis becomes erect in the middle of the night and ejaculation happens without any intentional stimulation. Though this can be messy, it is not an issue of sin. It is an issue of biology. For women, this might include a sexual dream that becomes arousing enough to lead to an orgasm. You may have felt the need to confess this as if it was sin. However, wet dreams and sexual dreams cannot be controlled, other than making sure you are not pursuing any erotica during the waking hours. Orgasms do happen organically and spontaneously. Though you can definitely share it with someone you feel close to, just to be open with any challenges that might be connected, it can be helpful to remember that, once again, God did an amazing job when He created the human body.

For the single and teen disciple, it is important to understand physiology so that that knowledge may help you understand where your hands should or should not go if you are pursuing purity in your romantic relationships. Young men, it is important for you to know that touching the region around your girlfriend's breasts or vulva could create sexual arousal, a response God intends for the marital relationship. Young women, touching your boyfriend's penis (or upper thigh) or laying up against him where your body touches his penis or your breasts press against him, will most likely create sexual arousal in your boyfriend, which again is a response that God intends between a wife and husband. There is an "appropriate time" for love to be arousing. Understanding physiology can then help you make godly choices about when those arousing touches should happen.

Remember, you are fearfully and wonderfully made, and yes, that includes your vulva and your penis. So treat those parts of your body and others' bodies with the special honor that God intends.

EXERCISE

Communication Exercise About Anatomy

After reading this chapter, take some time to speak with a trusted friend. Consider using these questions to guide your time together.

1. What did you learn about sexual anatomy that you did not know before?
2. When you consider arousal, what beliefs do you have about your response to arousal?
3. How can you practically apply your beliefs to your experience of arousal?
4. What kinds of questions do you still have about how your body works and how sexuality works?

CHAPTER 9

PURITY AND HOLINESS

"How can a young man keep his way pure?
By living according to Your word."

PSALM 119:9

Many of us grew up hearing a lot of different messages about sex. For some, there was no message—only silence. But silence about sex can communicate a certain message. If you grew up in a family that didn't talk about sex much, you might have gotten the message that sex was shameful or that it's taboo to talk about sex. If you experienced molestation or were surrounded by a confusing array of sexual examples, you may have felt that sex was dirty or hidden, or that there are no boundaries at all to the kind of sex you can engage in. Within my family, I (Tim) had an array of inappropriate sexual examples from family members and my church community. I also was exposed at an early age to an array of sexual media, such as Playboy and Penthouse magazines and an outdoor XXX theater near my home where we could sneak in to see through the trees. These kinds of influences are confusing for a growing child who is trying to figure out what to do with this thing called sex. We often get a whole different set of messages from church. These usually boil down to sex as a list of don'ts—don't get pregnant, don't wear that, don't watch that.

So for many of us, when the word *purity* gets brought up, it is either not a positive word, or it is confusing. And staying pure, having sexual integrity, can often sound more like a deprivation than a privilege and a benefit. As those who believe the Bible to be the standard for our sexual ethic, how are we to view and practice purity? How do we live out our sexuality by the biblical sexual ethic? By sexual ethic, we mean the set of values and beliefs a person may have that guides what they choose to do sexually.

There are many kinds of answers about how to view and practice purity that can be very unfulfilling. "True Love Waits." That sounds great, and it also sounds like an old love story movie title. Many times, faithful Christians get tired of hearing the same old answers—old answers that are sometimes given little theological support. "Those who have sex before marriage get STDs and end up divorced." If you try to use this one to convince someone to remain pure, they will have plenty of time to shoot holes in it. The reality is there are innumerable people who have had sex before marriage who have no STDs. And many couples who get married, those who stay married and those who divorce, had sex before marriage. This does not at all mean we should not strive for honoring God's plan to wait to engage sexually until marriage. However, it is important to emphasize that using trite, empty, or tired arguments usually leads to dismissal or avoidance of dealing with some of the real issues beneath the choice to engage sexually.

In our walk as disciples of Jesus, we are all called to be disciplined. "For God did not give us a spirit of timidity, but a spirit of power, of love, and of self-discipline" (2 Timothy 1:7). Much of pursuing sexual integrity and holiness is a reflection of sexual discipline. "Submit yourselves, then, to God. Resist the devil, and he will flee from you. Come near to God and he will come near to you" (James 4:7-8). We have to put on the armor of God (Ephesians 6:10-18) in order to live the life of peace God intends, free from the damage of sexual sin (Romans 8:6). But how do we do that? Let's examine that question.

Scriptural Foundation for Purity

There are over 70 references to sexual sin in the Bible, and sexual sin is the chief area of sin and brokenness in the Bible. However, in order to build a foundation for purity, studying those Scriptures about sin is just part of the battle. We must also study what we are aiming for. Purity. Here are a few scriptures to get us started:

> "Therefore, since we have these promises, dear friends, let us purify ourselves from everything that contaminates body and spirit, perfecting holiness out of reverence for God."
>
> 2 CORINTHIANS 7:1

> "It is God's will that you should be sanctified: that you should avoid sexual immorality; that each of you should learn to control your own body in a way that is holy and honorable."
>
> 1 THESSALONIANS 4:3-4

> "And this is my prayer: that your love may abound more and more in knowledge and depth of insight, so that you may be able to discern what is best and may be pure and blameless for the day of Christ."
>
> PHILIPPIANS 1:10

It may first be helpful to understand the words used in these scriptures. In the Greek, the term for *purify yourselves* and *sanctified* is the word *katharos* meaning clean and unstained. This word is usually associated with a clean heart, conscience, character, and religion, or a clean item such as gold or linen. *Holiness* is the Greek word *hagnos*, which means free from defilement, holy, sacred, chaste, unadulterated, uncontaminated, unspoiled, separated to God. This word is translated in various ways as free from sin, innocent, and pure. The word *honorable* in the Greek is *time* which means price, honor, perceived value and worth, to esteem and respect. In Philippians, we find a unique term, *eilikrines,* which means unalloyed, unmixed, sincere, and judged by sunlight. What a wonderful word, where the sunlight of divine clarity can give true insight and discernment. These words describe the beauty of purity.

We need to embrace the meanings of these various words. Sacred. Unstained. Unspoiled. Innocent. Of value and worth. Full of sunlight. If we had to choose between drinking contaminated water and drinking purified water, there is no question that we would say purified water is the better choice. One of the benefits of living in certain nations is the availability of pure drinking water. We can be grateful to live in a country where that is what we have. However, with sex, staying pure can seem like we are getting the least preferable, less exciting choice. We can often fail to see it as a benefit, as a gift, as a joy.

When we have met with groups of singles, teenagers, or college students to talk about purity, we usually ask them how they feel about the topic. Often, what we hear is, "Here we go again. Another lesson on how we need to protect the brothers/the sisters. Another lesson about not wearing short shorts and low-cut tops, not hugging too close. Another lesson about how we should run away from sex and not masturbate." Yes, these responses may be a reflection of a lack of hungering for righteousness (Matthew 5:6). However, we also have to face the fact that we can make pursuing purity a list of rules and regulations. And this is not God's intention.

Look at some of the other scriptures where God talks about purity:

"Each one of you know how to control his own body in holiness and honor."

1 THESSALONIANS 4:4

"Pursue righteousness, faith, love, and peace, along with those who call on the Lord from a pure heart."

2 TIMOTHY 2:22

"Finally, brothers, whatever is true, whatever is honorable, whatever is just, whatever is pure ... think about these things."

PHILIPPIANS 4:8

"To the pure, all things are pure."

TITUS 1:15

"For the Lord God is a sun and shield; the Lord bestows favor and honor. No good thing does he withhold from those who walk uprightly."

PSALMS 84:11

"Blessed are the pure in heart, for they shall see God."

MATTHEW 5:8

"To the pure you show yourself pure."

PSALMS 18:26

"Everyone who has this hope fixed on Him purifies himself, just as He is pure."

1 JOHN 3:3

"Holy, innocent, undefiled."

HEBREWS 7:26

"Who may ascend into the hill of the LORD? And who may stand in His holy place? He who has clean hands and a pure heart."

PSALMS 24:3

God obviously views purity with very positive words: holy, undefiled, clean, hope, honorable, just. And purity is associated with very positive ideas and verbs: *see* God, *stand* in His holy place, *walk* uprightly, *hope fixed* on Him. There are specific verbs in these scriptures that are associated with a life of purity: ascend, stand, see, walk, control, pursue. The apostle Paul says in 1 Corinthians 9:27 that he beats his body (strictly disciplines it) to make it his slave. Because Paul has spent considerable time in the first letter to the Corinthians exhorting the Christians to flee sexual immorality, we can conclude that this reference to *beating his body* includes having the control to keep from sinning sexually. The Greek word for *control* (v.25, every athlete practices self-control) is definitely associated with how we manage our bodies sexually (1 Thessalonians 4:4). Surrounding these ideas of mastering sexual impulses is the shining goal of righteousness, holiness, and purity. Purity is not some depressing, grin-and-bear-it goal. It is a beautiful beacon. A beacon is both a warning and a cause for celebration. We should absolutely utilize God's word to warn us away from the lure of sexual immorality, but we should also celebrate the joy of standing upright in God's presence with pure consciences, bodies, and hearts—with clean hands and eyes set on Him. He is both a sun and shield. He gives us warmth and protects us. We need God for both of those things when it comes to the practice of purity. We need both the warmth of the sun and the shield against the storm. And, yes, purity is a practice. It is a continual choice to stand in God's holy place and walk up His hill, looking into the beauty of His face. In the world, the idea of purity, of deciding to live a life free from sexual involvement unless one is married, seems strange, repressed, and completely old-fashioned—or even backward. Peter said, "They think it strange that you do not jump with them into the same flood of dissipation" (1 Peter 4:4). For many, pursuing purity is strange and weird, even stupid. How dumb is it to go into marriage with no idea of whether you are sexually compatible? So what is a girl to do? How does a young man, or an older man for that matter, combat the negative view of purity, let alone hold to that conviction without actually being weird?

Motivation for Purity

> "Therefore, whatever you eat or drink, or whatever you do, do all
> for the glory of God."
>
> 1 CORINTHIANS 10:31

People are motivated to pursue purity for a number of different reasons. Those trying to stop doing pornography and masturbation may be looking to find freedom, to get rid of guilt, to feel better about themselves, to fix relationships they have damaged, or to avoid messing up future relationships. However, each of these motivations, though completely understandable, are still self-focused. For change to last, keeping your eyes focused on God and wanting to bring Him glory in how you live gets to the heart of why we deal with all sin in our lives. When Gideon was chosen to lead the Israelites in battle against the Midianites, the Lord told Gideon, "The people who are with you are too many for Me to give the Midianites into their hands, lest Israel claim glory for itself against Me, saying, 'My own hand has saved me'" (Judges 7:2). God makes it clear that He wants us to fight the battle, but He wants us to remember by whose hand we are saved. God does not want us to say boastfully, "Look at me. Look how I have battled to be pure. What a good example I am." Jeremiah 9:24 says, "Let him who boasts boast in this: that he understands and knows me." God calls us to boast in knowing Him, to give the glory to Him, to remember that He is the one who has given us the strength to change.

The goal for each disciple of Jesus is transformation—to be transformed into His image, to represent Him. "We all ... are being transformed into his image with ever-increasing glory, which comes from the Lord, who is the Spirit" (2 Corinthians 3:18). In order to be transformed, our heart must seek His glory. We do this by fixing our eyes on Jesus (Hebrews 12:2). Jesus is the radiance of God's glory (Hebrews 1:3), so if we put our eyes on Him, we will be looking at God's glory and we will be transformed. We mentioned earlier that we would all choose purified drinking water rather than contaminated drinking water. Jesus is the provider of that clean, pure water (John 4:14). Put your eyes there and ask Him for a drink.

Boundaries

For those of you striving to help others pursue purity, remember that pat answers can leave someone feeling like their challenges with remaining pure are trivial. "All you have to do is walk away." Those kinds of answers can make it sound like chastity, or pursuing purity, is easy. It isn't. However, support, direction, guidance, and healthy boundaries are absolutely vital to the process of maintaining a pure lifestyle.

So, what are some healthy boundaries to maintain purity? If you are dating, ask yourselves, have you had this conversation with your boyfriend or girlfriend? Have you talked together about what convictions, feelings, or beliefs you have around the physical part of the relationship? If you are not yet dating, what kind of convictions do you have now? Have you thought about it? Do you have scriptures to back up those thoughts and convictions? Do you have a clear plan of what you want in your future relationships? If you are a parent or mentor for someone engaged in, or contemplating, a relationship, what direction would you give them, and what is that founded on? These are all important things to think about before a relationship begins. Before emotion comes flooding in and possibly sends convictions out the window. We have included these questions at the end of the chapter to guide your own exploration and communication.

Some of you may have had strong beliefs about the sexual and physical boundaries you should have, but those boundaries have been crossed in many of your relationships. For some of you, you may have been involved with someone who violated you in some way and forced sexual touch or sex on you. Or you did not feel the freedom to say no—or felt you couldn't or shouldn't say no to them. Cliff and Joyce Penner convey an important point in their book *The Gift of Sex* where they emphasize that sex should be by invitation only. This is extremely important. It is not only that when someone says no, then the answer is no. The deeper level here is that unless someone has invited the other to have sex with them, or to touch them sexually, there is a very good chance that a violation could happen.

For others of you who willingly engaged in sex or sexual play, even though you had beliefs that you shouldn't, it may be important to ask yourself, "If I did have boundaries, especially if I communicated those boundaries, why did I allow others to trespass? Why did I back down or give in?"

When I (Jennifer) speak with young women about this, I ask them, "What led you to decide you were not worth enough to expect that your wishes should be respected? What stopped you from expecting the other to not only honor your wishes but also to seek them out?" I have asked these same questions of men. If you had strong convictions, have you had partners that have pressed against or questioned those convictions? Yes, we should each make good choices in aligning ourselves with those who hold the same convictions we have about purity and boundaries. However, it can be a growth-producing process to contemplate why we allow someone to cause us to go against the voice in our head, against our own integrity. You have integrity. It might be a new decision on your part to expect respect and to expect that someone would honor and uphold your integrity.

Treat Them with Special Honor

One of our favorite passages to use when teaching about purity is one that is often overlooked. Paul, in 1 Corinthians 12:23, exhorts Christians to treat everyone in the body of Christ with honor, especially those in the church who have a role we might consider less important. He uses the physical body to make this point. "The parts we think are less honorable we treat with special honor. And the parts that are unpresentable are treated with special modesty." We apply this scripture rightly to the spiritual body of Christ, but sometimes don't realize what God is also saying here about the physical body. We have unpresentable parts. What are they? When we ask this question to groups, we commonly get the same answers. The parts of our body that are unpresentable are the penis, the vulva, the buttocks, and the breasts. So how does God say we are to treat those parts of our body? *With special honor!*

This is such an important point. Being modest, living a pure life, is not just a matter of "Don't wear that" and "Cover that up." These words are commonly said to a Christian woman in regards to those parts of her body. Sometimes, those commands are given to a young girl or a woman in an irritated or even condemning tone. If you are the one having that conversation with a woman when you have become concerned with her lack of modesty or her choice in clothing, think about the tone with which you want to have that conversation.

Let's take a careful look at what the meaning of these different words tells us. God says our bodies are fearfully and wonderfully made (Psalms 139:14). These words have been described in detail in the chapter five, *Body Image*. When you approach someone, make sure that is your mindset. God did an incredible job when He made the human body. It is a beautiful work of art. When you consider your own choices about how to dress, remember with reverence and awe the amazing work of creation God did in making your body. Then, when you consider what to put on that body, remember, God says that these parts of your body—your breasts, your buttocks, your vulva, and yes, the male penis—are not to be presented openly to others in public. Rather, like rare jewels and precious gems, they are to be kept in safety and treated with special honor.

The term in the Greek for *special honor* is *euschemosune time* (external charm special) and for *special modesty* are *euschemosune perissos* (modesty special). We know that *time* means something of incredible value. *Euschemosune* means decorum, comeliness, seemliness, modesty, good outward form; where something that is of high or prominent position is treated with proper respect. *Perissos* means greater, more, abounding, abundant, excessive, exceeding, and beyond what is expected. God wants us to treat these parts—those that He says should not be presented publicly—with an extraordinary, abundant, over-the-top amount of respect, value, and decorum. So covering up, dressing modestly, should never be, in *any way*, a practice of embarrassment or shame but rather a choice that shows great honor and value to things that are precious and beyond worth.

For men, remember this incredible passage. How are you doing treating those parts of women's bodies? Are you looking at them in ways that are not modest, that do not show respect and honor to that woman? Are you treating women's vaginas, vulvas, buttocks, and breasts with abundant value and respect? Do you regard the intimate parts of a woman's body as sacred ground, a place of holiness and honor reserved for marriage? Do your eyes, thoughts and conversation reflect the value and respect a woman deserves as God's daughter? If you engage in taking a lingering second look at a woman's bottom, if your gaze goes to her breasts rather than her eyes, are you treating those parts of her body as God would have you treat them? It is incredibly true that in most of today's society, these parts have been displayed in full view on every television screen and billboard. They are displayed before you by your female coworkers and by other women as you walk along the street. Sometimes they are displayed even as you stand next to a young girl or woman at church. However, God's call to you does not change. Even if the media is dishonoring, even if a woman does not treat her own body with respect, you are called to. This can be a particular challenge if you have been involved with pornography. You may have to work hard at training your eyes and your mind toward reclaiming the depth of honor God gives to the parts of the body that have been extremely objectified— not only in pornographic video and pictures, but in many other forms of media. These same teachings would also apply to the penis and the male buttocks. Remember, a man's penis is fearfully and wonderfully made (Psalm 139:14). It is to be treated with the same level of honor, value, and respect. Ladies, how are you doing in treating these parts of a man's body? Do you excuse yourself from the conversation when friends make coarse comments about men's bodies or their sexuality? Do your eyes, thoughts and conversation reflect the value and respect a man deserves as God's son?

When our children were young, we taught them the Scripture in Psalm 139 about their bodies. At an early age, children become very interested in exploring their genitals. We spoke with our children about how these parts of their body were incredibly special and, therefore, were not toys to be played with or to be displayed. These special parts were only to be displayed and sexually enjoyed when they were in a married relationship with their spouse.

We are fearfully and wonderfully made. Treat your body as a temple. And treat those parts of your body that you do not present publicly as precious and of great value.

PRACTICAL DIRECTION

In the following sections, we are going to provide some practical suggestions for pursuing purity and overcoming the pulls to impurity. We want to emphasize that this section is not just meant for men. Both men and women struggle with remaining pure. We need to support both our brothers and our sisters in their pursuit.

Where Are You Lurking?

Job says, "I made a covenant with my eyes; why then would I look lustfully at a young woman?" Job also talks about, if he was "enticed by a woman" or "lurking at his neighbor's door," how could he expect his own wife to be faithful. There are several helpful parts about how Job speaks here. Ask yourself, have you made a covenant with your eyes? This word *covenant* in the Hebrew is *berith*, meaning a treaty or an alliance. One of the first steps to keeping our thoughts and eyes where they need to be, not lurking where we should not, is by making an alliance with those thoughts and eyes. Make a treaty with them. Come up with an agreement between your heart, mind, and eyes about where you're going to put them and what kinds of thoughts you're going to allow to develop from what they see. Have you made that alliance? That is a good place to start.

A part of that covenant is getting rid of the junk. Do you still purchase those romance novels to get that kick, that sexual thrill? Do you still watch those movies to feel that sexual pull? Do you still have that website in your favorites? Do you still walk by that venue you have visited before? Where are you lurking? In order to keep your eyes and heart faithful, you may have to make some radical decisions about what to put before them.

Secondly, men, how do you view women? Women, how do you view men? How do you view their bodies? Do you look at them with lust, or do you look at them as a whole person. Douglas Rosenau, in his book *The Celebration of Sex*, has a wonderful recommendation for men (which can also be applied to women) who struggle with lustfully taking a second look at a woman or at an advertisement or billboard. He calls this *3-D sexuality*. Rosenau states, "When you are at the mall and notice an attractive woman, look at her face and notice if she is tired. Observe the packages she is carrying and think, *I bet she's a great mom*. Make the woman a person and give her a life." For women, this might apply when a man brazenly jogs down your street shirtless. Look at his face, while reminding yourself how God sees him. Remind yourself that he is a child of God and say a short prayer for him.

Rosenau also suggests that men look at the less common but very feminine features of a woman's body like her hands, her smile, and her ways of gesturing. Ask yourself if you would want someone looking at your daughter or future wife the way you are tempted to look at her. Pray for her and her relationship with God. He mentions thinking through who this person is. They are someone's daughter or son. Perhaps they are a student or they have a job. They are someone's friend. Someone's child. Someone's parent. When you focus on the sexual parts of their body that draw your eye, when you imagine sexual scenes, that man, that woman becomes an object and a non-person. So make them into a person. Remember they were a child and have a past. They have a life and they are special and important to God.

Masturbation and Pornography

The pursuit of purity often includes how to respond to the pull to masturbate or view pornography. We address this in greater detail in chapter ten, but want to address here the underlying pursuit of purity and how that influences the pull toward these practices.

There are certain common times when people are tempted to masturbate and use pornography. These are often late at night, when someone is feeling stressed or sad, when they are bored, or when they feel or are alone. It isn't uncommon for someone to say they got home after an exhausting week and wanted to do something to relax. Because their pattern has been to go to something sexual when they are feeling that way, there often is no consideration that their real need may be something else.

When you need rest, relaxation, and relief from stress, you may seek to fill it with something entertaining or fun. Pursuing something sexual often becomes an automatic way to fulfill that need for fun. However, there can be such a greater sense of fulfillment if you choose differently. When a wave of desire washes through you, pulling you towards a sexual behavior—getting on the computer and scrolling through pornography or reading or watching something and masturbating—instead pursue another way to fulfill that need. Instead of pursuing something sexual, do something fun with a close friend, play basketball with someone you are reaching out to, go somewhere beautiful that fills the soul, share heartfelt feelings with a close confidante, or reach out for a compliment or hug from a real friend.

Recognizing the underlying need and responding righteously to the pulls to masturbate and do pornography is an incredibly important part of pursuing purity. We have therefore included an entire section on them. See chapter ten, *Masturbation and Pornography*.

Fill the House with Good Things

The plans above for how to ride the wave go along with what the Scriptures teach. Jesus taught that "when an impure spirit comes out of a person, it goes through arid places seeking rest and does not find it. Then it says, 'I will return to the house I left.' When it arrives, it finds the house unoccupied, swept clean and put in order. Then it goes and takes with it seven other spirits more wicked than itself, and they go in and live there. And the final condition of that person is worse than the first" (Matthew 12:43-45). You have shoved the evil spirit of impurity out of your life. However, we know Satan is not done. He's gonna come back and try to take root again. Jesus lets us know that it is not enough to just sweep the house clean. We need to fill that house with good things. When I (Jennifer) work with those involved in sexual addiction, I guide them through a process of figuring out what they will use to fill their house. When they are pulled toward pornography and/or masturbation, they need to make a plan ahead of time for what they are going to reach for instead.

So, what will you fill your house with? There are so many possibilities which hold different appeal for each person. What kind of new, enriching hobby can you pursue? How are your close friendships going? Do you need to invest in some relationships in order to have a safe haven to go to when you need to talk? How are you doing in serving others? What is a spiritual challenge you want to pursue: learning Old and New Testament history, memorizing Scripture, aiding someone in learning the Bible, or doing an in-depth study of a particular topic? What kind of art draws you (music, poetry, photography, painting)? Have you wanted to pursue gardening or a building project?

When I (Tim) travel for my work, I have to have a specific plan in order to maintain my purity. I keep my time with God active by reading

His Word and praying, and I find that speaking with my wife daily is important for my heart and motivation. I also plan enjoyable activities with disciples in the city I am visiting as well as with coworkers. Each of these things can seem like a panacea, like a snake-oil remedy for a serious illness. However, if you do not have a plan on how to fill your house up with life-giving joy and fun, that long-term pattern of turning to something sexual will merely return.

As it is sometimes stated, "Real sexual integrity is not about what you aren't doing; it's about what you are doing." This includes not only filling your house with good things, but also figuring out some of the underlying issues that lead you to using sexual means to relieve boredom, stress, anger, and sadness. People often pursue sexual activities to relieve these emotions. It is vital in the process of pursuing purity to recognize the underlying anxiety that may be driving the sexual behavior.

In Alcoholics Anonymous, they emphasize that stopping drinking for some becomes just a white knuckling experience; when someone grits their teeth to keep themselves from drinking. However, those involved in solid recovery will point out that if someone stops themselves from drinking through white knuckling or gritting their teeth, and does not address what lies underneath the pull to drink (i.e., the anxiety they are feeling), their process of recovery and sobriety will be at risk. Those who want to have ongoing victory must deal with the underlying emotional issues that may have led to a pattern of use in order to have lifelong recovery. And so they must recognize the pulls and needs and then intentionally fill up their house with good stuff.

Response to Sexual Cues

"I don't think it is higher testosterone or our sexual natures that always make us more sexually aroused. Rather, it is our poor self-discipline of the environmental sexual cues."

Rosenau, *The Celebration of Sex*

Ask yourself how you're doing with disciplining yourself on how you respond to the many sexual cues out there. You may not be able to stop the initial sexual stimulation (the thought, the picture), but you can choose to tell that thought that it cannot just stay for a visit. Guy Hammond, in *Tempt Away*, shares a hilarious example. When his mind wants to go somewhere he does not want it to go, he initially distracts himself by doing the Steve Martin "wild and crazy guy" move, shaking his arms and legs and body. You might think that's crazy and silly, but the reality for some is, whatever it takes! Get silly. Be humble, and do whatever you need to do to ride that initial response to a sexual cue and come out on the other side not having given in to the pull.

Pursuing sexual activities can involve two different motivators: satiation and excitation. We spoke about satiation earlier, the desire to satiate uncomfortable emotions like sadness, anxiety, and anger, by pursuing something sexual. Excitation is pursuing something sexual because of how thrilling and exciting we think it will be. This is the excitement of the chase, the pursuit of the high. The thrill of looking for or responding to something new. When that sexual cue happens, when you can feel your heart rate pick up and you can feel the draw to respond to the exciting call, it is important that you think through ahead of time what you are going to do. Have a specific plan for something exciting you can do that does not include sex. Let's talk about some components of that plan.

Pre-work

To experience success to sexual cues, there is often some pre-work to do before the pull even walks in the room. Pre-work is calling up that friend and saying that you're going to have an evening downtown, or at the beach, or alone and bored, and you want them to know that it could be a tempting time for you. Pre-work is making sure that you have a good work-out or a special prayer time planned to ease anxiety and tension so that the peace of God can guard your heart. If you are not setting yourself up for success ahead of time, when the pull comes, the allure of it can overtake you quickly. So again, filling up the house is not just about what to do when you feel the pulls. It is also about what to do beforehand to lessen the power of that pull.

Openness

This is Number One. Who are you open with? Do your friends know your struggle? Are you meeting with a support group to find ways to overcome? Yes, God knows, but until you bring that challenge into the light, Satan can have a heyday. "If we claim to have fellowship with Him and yet walk in the darkness, we lie and do not live by the truth. But if we walk in the light, as He is in the light, we have fellowship with one another, and the blood of Jesus, His Son, purifies us from all sin" (1 John 1:6-7). What an incredible passage. When you are open, when you come into the light, you have fellowship with one another. The word *fellowship* here is *koinonia*, a partnership, a contributory help, a participation and sharing in common with, a spiritual community. God says that when we share openly, not only do we get the support of spiritual partners to hold up our arms in the battle, we also are purified by the blood of Jesus. Purified and made clean. By blood. By the blood of an innocent man. How amazing is that? Pursue openness. The benefits are eternal, daily, and real.

The spiritual disciplines are challenging. Daily prayer. Daily reading of the Word. Fasting. Daily fellowship and encouragement. Daily worship. The sexual disciplines are equally challenging and vital and include filling up the house with good things.

Helping Others

You may not only be in pursuit of your own holiness, but you may also have the privilege of helping others. How does one go about that? One participant of a workshop we did asked, "What is the best way to answer single sisters [and brothers] who 'confess' being impure and feel guilty about it? How can we help stop this habit or behavior of masturbation when so many confess doing it? What to say?"

There is no question that the Scriptures instruct us to teach and admonish one another. However, in the area of sexuality, disciples of Jesus can have a strong aversion to asking sexual questions. Often, people either avoid the topic altogether or they deal with it in a harsh or shaming way. How can we treat one another with honor and dignity while probing into such a personal area?

It's helpful to understand that our aversion to doing this permeates our society. In his 1986 dissenting opinion, Supreme Court Justice John Harry Blackmun states, "How a person engages in sex should be irrelevant as a matter of state law. Sexual intimacy is a sensitive, key relationship of human existence and the development of human personality. In a diverse nation such as ours, we must preserve the individual freedom to choose, and not imply that there are any 'right' ways of conducting relationships." This may be a valid argument for a government, but how is a disciple of Jesus to respond. For disciples committed to *one another* relationships and to helping present one another fully mature in Christ (Colossians 1:28), if you ask about someone's sexual activities, it can feel like you're sticking your nose into someone's bedroom and invading their right to privacy. We live in a world that upholds individual liberty, and deciding to get involved in one another's lives in these areas can seem counter to all we hold dear.

However, counter to the individualism of our culture, it is vital for the follower of Jesus to remember what his or her role is in the body of Christ. We are called to help one another and carry each other's burdens. "Brothers and sisters, if someone is caught in a sin, you who live by the Spirit should restore that person gently ... Carry each other's burdens, and in this way you will fulfill the law of Christ" (Galatians 6:1). If someone reads this scripture without understanding the intent of the passage, it might seem like God would expect us to peer into each other's windows in order to catch someone doing something illicit. Rather, the passage here lets us know that we are our brother's keeper in that we are responsible to care and be involved enough in each other's lives so that we can see when someone has been ensnared by sin (2 Timothy 2:25) and may need a hand in being reconciled to God (2 Corinthians 5:18-20). So, in love, peer into each other's lives. With respect, honesty, and directness ("rebuke your neighbor frankly" in Leviticus 19:17), take the time to ask the questions that might save your sister or brother's soul.

If you are one who tends to charge in with little love or gentleness, go to those who shepherd God's people and learn from them. We both have benefitted immensely through the years from the amazing wisdom of those who are elders and leaders in God's family. These men and women have guided our words and hearts as we have striven to stay pure ourselves and to help those involved in sexual sin. They have helped us see our own sin and self-righteousness—sometimes with a gentle word, sometimes with a direct rebuke. If you are in a role of helping and leading others, continually put yourself under these kinds of spiritual shepherds so that you can have better discernment. You will find guidance for when to "warn those who are idle and disruptive, encourage the disheartened, help the weak, be patient with everyone" (1 Thessalonians 5:14). You will understand when to "gently instruct in the hope that God will grant them repentance leading them to a knowledge of the truth and that they will come to their senses and escape from the trap of the devil, who has taken them captive to do his will" (2 Timothy 2:25). For those of us who tend more toward harsh and unloving tones, it is vital to hear the words used in these passages: warn, encourage, help, be patient, gently instruct. There is a time and place for rebuke and church discipline (Luke 17:3, Matthew 18:15-17, 2 Timothy 3:16). Seek counsel yourself as you seek to counsel others so that you can rightly handle the word of truth and be an instrument in God's hands to restore your sister or brother.

We end this chapter with some words from our brother Dave Eastman. "What is God's desire for you, single brother/sister? That you and one special person develop a great friendship, enjoy a pure relationship, enter marriage enjoying the full blessing of God, enjoy the greatest possible sexual relationship, and walk through life as soul mates, helping one another to make it all the way to heaven. That's the fairy tale. And thousands of couples in our fellowship worldwide have lived it to this day. Don't allow your hormonal fantasies, the fables of Hollywood, and the myths of Satan to rob you of that fairy tale in your own life."

If you have already had some deep falls, remember, it is never too late to pursue God's redemption of sexuality. As the Bible says, "Today is the day of salvation" (2 Corinthians 6:2). What truly matters is the decisions you make today. Take some time to go back through this discussion, and decide where God would have you start *today*. If you are in a relationship that has wandered from God's standards, bring your struggles into God's restorative, atoning light (confessing to others who will graciously help you) and together recommit to His beautiful plan of purity. Remember, the Christian "fairy tale" isn't so much about perfection as it is about pursuit. Pursue purity today, and it will bless you with a strong foundation for an incredible future.

EXERCISE

Foundations for Purity

Spend some time with the questions below, journaling your thoughts. After you think and pray through this exercise, spend time with someone you trust and share your answers.

1. What are your convictions about purity? What scriptures would you use to explain those convictions?
2. What are your beliefs about masturbation? What are your beliefs about pornography?
3. If you put together a personal plan for purity, what would you include in that?
4. If you are dating, have you talked together about what your boundaries are in your physical relationship?

5. What kind of convictions, feelings, or beliefs do you have about the physical part of the relationship for a dating couple? An engaged couple? Identify and write out Scriptures to back up your thoughts and convictions?

6. If you are a parent or mentor for someone engaged in, or contemplating, a relationship, what direction would you give them, and what is that founded on (i.e., Scriptures, experience)?

CHAPTER 10

MASTURBATION AND
PORNOGRAPHY

W hy a whole chapter dedicated to masturbation and pornography? Without question, in our world today, one of the most difficult challenges for Christians who pursue purity is how to overcome the temptation to masturbate and view pornography. You may be reading this and saying, "Why are these even in the same chapter? Clearly pornography is wrong. But masturbation? Isn't it natural? Isn't it common? And besides, I've tried to change that so many times and it just isn't possible."

There are many different thoughts about masturbation, both within the Christian community and within the church. You have one camp that says masturbation is a natural response and that when sexual urges build up, there may be a need to release the sexual tension. So if someone habitually brings himself or herself to orgasm, but no other person is involved in their mind, then this would not be sin. This is an understandable argument, since we know that Jesus clearly teaches that we should not look at someone with lust and that lust is the same as adultery (Matthew 5:28). Others might say that any kind of sexual self-touch or masturbation is sex outside of the marriage bed and, therefore, sin. What is a disciple of Jesus to think?

To answer these vexing questions, it is important to consider the Bible's overarching view of sex. If you skipped ahead to this chapter, go back and read what the Bible says about sex (chapter one). There is a whole section on God's overall plan for sexuality. Remember, God guards and guides our sexuality. He does put healthy boundaries around sex, most likely because of the greater damage sexual sin can do. "He who sins sexually sins against his own body" (1 Corinthians 6:18). So what should our boundaries be?

A great place to start is to use the larger picture to seek answers to your questions. For instance, you might ask, "What exactly does the Bible say about masturbation?" Well, the truth is, absolutely nothing. The practice of masturbation is not addressed directly in Scripture. It is here where we need to remind ourselves of how God views sexuality overall. If you consider God's overarching plan for sexuality in the Bible, it is clear that sex is not only about the sexual act of sexual stimulation to orgasm. The Biblical examples of sex involve an intimate connection and the knowing that occurs between two (married) people engaged in godly sexual intimacy. The question then arises, where would individual masturbation fit? If it is not part of an intimate, knowing marital relationship, then does masturbation fit within the overarching view of sex in the Bible? We would suggest no.

Can we say, "Masturbation is sin?" This is a bit of a thornier question. As we have mentioned, there is no scripture verse that explicitly states that masturbation is a sin. Please understand that we are not saying that there is no sin involved in the practice of masturbation. However, what we are emphasizing is that each sexual choice we make must be governed by God's overarching purpose and plan for sex. Does this practice, in whatever fashion we engage in it, create connection and intimacy and knowing between two people bound together in a covenant relationship of marriage?

The other perspective we encourage disciples of Jesus to take is to examine the potential fruit of choosing to engage in a certain sexual practice (Matthew 7:17-20). Let's say you have a background of masturbating or pornography, a practice in which you believe God does not want you to engage because pornography includes other people, which Scripture clearly teaches against (Matthew 5:28). Even if you are seeking to masturbate without impure thoughts, you are still vulnerable to re-engaging in using pornography or fantasizing while masturbating, practices you know are wrong. The very practice of masturbation can trigger an old rut (more in a moment). Engaging in masturbation clearly becomes a "hint of sexual immorality" (Ephesians 5:3) or a "foothold" (Ephesians 4:27) for this individual. The fruit of this choice does not bring God's intended benefit.

Often individuals will share that they use masturbation to lower their anxiety levels, or that when they do not masturbate, their anxiety levels are higher. On the Internet, it's easy to find sites that not only support masturbation, but also list many physical and mental health benefits. Articles claim that it helps prevent cancer (especially prostate cancer), it helps keep the penile tissues and structure from having difficulties with erection (other research will claim the exact opposite), it boosts the person's mood and helps alleviate depression, and it aids in healthy blood flow. The month of May has even been declared "national masturbation month."

Note that the conclusions in these articles are drawn from research on the benefits of sex. For instance, research (primarily done on rats) has shown that orgasm raises levels of oxytocin, a hormone that is believed to facilitate the response to fear and anxiety. Authors use this research to then claim that lack of sex causes greater challenges with fear and anxiety. However, in the research community (of which Jennifer is a part), it would be considered incredibly poor research to make a claim that because a behavior causes something, then a lack of that behavior causes a deficit. This kind of approach can leave out the incredible number of ways that individuals choose to manage their fear and anxiety without using sex to cope. Masturbation leaves you emptier than when you began. It highlights the lack of focus on giving to the other that fills godly sexuality.

Remember, God's wisdom is foolishness to the world. Consider what you are using to help you make the decision whether to engage in masturbation. Ask yourself, other than looking on WebMD, are you seeking the advice of those over you in the Lord? Have you asked direction from those who are examples of faith? (Hebrews 13:7). God calls us to consult advisers who are men and women of faith and spiritual standing. Ask yourself… *Who are my advisers?*

Myths about Masturbation

In your quest for purity, you'll also want to be careful to separate myth from truth. We want to share a few of the myths out there about masturbation:

1. You won't be able to perform sexually when you're married.
2. It will make you blind (or some other serious illness).
3. If you masturbate, you *will* become sexually addicted.
4. You will get cancer if you don't ejaculate regularly.
5. When someone gets married, since they are having sex, they will no longer be interested in or be drawn to masturbation (or pornography).
6. There are no negative effects if you do not fantasize while masturbating.

Here is our attempt at addressing some of these possible myths:

#1 and #2. "Masturbation makes you blind" is a very old myth that we no longer hold to in our culture. In its heyday, this belief was written about in books, magazines, and medical journals as if it were truth. It obviously isn't since the 50-90 percent (depending on which study you read) of the male population are not walking around blind. Scare tactics get outed eventually. The problem with the statement that masturbation will cause problems with sexual functioning is that, though this is true for some, and quite possibly true for many, it is not absolutely true for all. Turning a myth into a warning does not help any argument.

Have researchers found that masturbation causes sexual functioning problems? Yes. Does this apply to everyone? Obviously not. But it does make you think twice. I (Tim) stopped using Rogaine when I found out it could cause problems with sexual functioning. Don't want nothin' messing with that. For Jennifer, these kinds of issues do come up in her professional work as a sexual counselor. Men who masturbate regularly have cited problems with obtaining an erection because the vagina does not provide the same level of friction as the hand. Women who masturbate find that their spouse just cannot provide the same kind of stimulation their hand or something else can. Though the blanket statement is a myth, the concern is valid.

#3. Though masturbation does not automatically cause addiction, most sexual addicts experiment first with masturbation, which then leads to increasing levels of pornography. Also, many sexual addicts engage in a proportionally high amount of masturbation. It is true that everyone who smokes marijuana will not become a meth and heroin addict; however, almost every meth and heroin addict began with marijuana. Though it never helps a debate to make false, exaggerated claims, it is always important to discover if there is any grain of truth behind those claims.

#4. Researchers have claimed that lack of orgasm, or lack of expelling semen, causes prostate cancer, lowers the immune system response, and lowers the quality of sperm that is ejaculated. There are also claims that masturbation helps with cramping and pain during menstruation, aids fertility, and keeps a woman's vulvar tissues healthy by keeping those tissues from atrophying (becoming dried up and stiff). Or, as it is claimed on the Internet, "use it or lose it." It is important to know that most of these studies (other than results for pain relief in women) have a number of problems: contradictory findings, poor research methodology, and a number of confounding variables (the studies do not do a good job of figuring out if it is eating red meat or masturbating that helps). There is no question that sex can have many health benefits. However, claiming that not having sex and not masturbating has health deficits is a questionable claim with little solid research to back it up. Also, it is not biblically sound reasoning to say that just because something makes us feel better physically does not mean it is best for our soul and spirit.

#5. As to whether the desire to masturbate (or view pornography) is lower once someone is married, most men report that this is true at the beginning of marriage (sometimes only the very beginning), but that if these habits were regular before marriage, they often not only return but continue to expand in marriage. In other words, marriage is not the cure. Genuinely embracing the pursuit of holiness, whether someone is married or single, is the cure and is the plan that God lays out in His Word.

#6. Other than the answers we have already given, we will leave this one for the advisers in your life. Ask the men and women of faith in your life, the trusted spiritual advisers who are spiritual examples, and the elders and elders' wives in your church, whether it plays out in real life that there are no negatives that result from masturbating without fantasizing. The question to ask here might be, though something could be permissible, is it beneficial and does it build up (1 Corinthians 6:12)?

Truths about Masturbation

1. Masturbating to sexual release (orgasm) does flood the brain with pleasurable feelings due to an increase of dopamine, oxytocin, and other pleasurable sex hormones.
2. There are no scripture verses that say masturbation is a sin.
3. The penis and vulva can become accustomed or conditioned to receiving a certain type of pressure and type of touch or grip in order to achieve orgasm.

4. Regular masturbation can lead to a kind of "tolerance" where greater, firmer, more idiosyncratic (unusual) touch is needed— or increasingly more varied forms of fantasy or pornography may be needed to produce enough arousal.

It is absolutely true that orgasm, whether it is induced by masturbation, intercourse, or some other stimulation, causes intense feelings of pleasure. Orgasm does increase oxytocin (the hormone that creates feelings of comfort, peace, and joy) and dopamine (the reward hormone that tells the body "this is very good"). These are the same chemicals that are released during sexual intercourse or when someone engages in various addictions such as drug use and gambling. The release of the chemicals in association with masturbation is actually what makes stopping masturbation and doing pornography so difficult.

It is true that there is no specific scripture that says masturbation is a sin. However, that does not mean that masturbation might not be "missing the mark" of God's holiness. Also, becoming accustomed to a particular kind of friction or touch from your own hand can condition your brain and body to that level and type of sexual stimulation. This can become particularly problematic if you get married and the kind of touch provided by your partner does not match your pre-marriage habits of self-stimulation. Either your spouse doesn't caress you the way you touched yourself (penis or vagina) or, guys, your wife's vagina is not as tight as your own hand's pressure. As Mark Laaser says, becoming dependent on ever-increasing pressure and intensity (tolerance) can make it difficult to be sexually responsive to the stimulation coming from sexual intercourse with a partner. This kind of conditioning has left some men and women frustrated because they cannot enjoy their sexual relationship with their spouse as they envisioned. Their sexual response has become wired to their own hand rather than their spouse's touch and body.

You might be tempted to despair if this is your situation. What is encouraging is that pursuing God, making a renewed commitment to holiness, and pursuing sexuality as God intends can help us re-experience, or perhaps even rewire, those brain circuits that may have gotten entrenched in a particular pattern. As a single, now is the time for you to re-educate your brain through abstinence from masturbation bolstered by new convictions. Holiness has rich benefits (Romans 6:22) and sets a guard against Satan's schemes to hijack your desires.

Pornography: The Great Hijacker

Mark Laaser, a therapist and sexual addiction specialist, explains that the human brain can be chemically hijacked by pornography. In this scenario, the brain could become neurochemically dependent on (or tolerant of) pornography and could, therefore, begin to crave (possibly due to withdrawal) the chemical rush created by viewing pornography. Laaser says that masturbation and particularly masturbation with pornography, becomes like sexual cocaine for the body and that indulging in that can be like playing with chemical fire. Though there is little scientific evidence to establish these claims without reservation, many individuals share that this is what they have experienced—that it becomes increasingly difficult to achieve the ability to enjoy sex with a partner when they have been involved with pornography.

On a long, across-America camping trip, we visited the Oregon Ruts. If you have never seen these, they are quite amazing. During the days

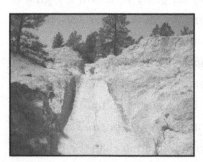

of wagon travel, as those going west took the Oregon Trail, they crossed over hard sandstone and granite territory. The ruts created by the thousands upon thousands of wagon wheels have created entrenched, deep grooves in the landscape.

Picturing this can be a very helpful way of understanding how the brain works. We take a certain action on a regular basis and the brain begins to create a pathway that becomes familiar with use. Over time, that pathway can become so entrenched and the brain circuitry response so automatic, that those patterns of behavior have a very difficult time going along any other direction. How many times do we accidently drive down a road and turn a certain direction automatically, without thinking, when we actually meant to go somewhere else? Behavioral patterns, both those that are beneficial and those that are not, can change but it often takes forging a new pathway, pushing against the ingrained ruts, and doing this over and over until a new way of travelling becomes the norm.

Many of us think that once we get married, all of our purity struggles will cease to exist. We might say to ourselves, "We're going to be having all that sex, so I'll never be tempted again." After marriage, I (Tim) did not struggle with my purity for several years as long as I was not traveling for my job. When I had to travel, I found staying pure very challenging. I learned some painful lessons early on and after that, as I travelled, I learned to fill my nights with work, going to the midweek church service in that area, reaching out to a co-worker, seeing a movie, or exploring the local area for its history. Whenever coworkers came along, I called many of these "team building events." I have worked hard at creating new pathways, new ruts.

You may need to look at some of the practicals in the *Purity and Holiness* chapter to overcome the habit of masturbation and pornography. And like we mentioned, in order to create those new habits, those new pathways, you may need to examine the non-sexual needs that are clamoring for your attention. You might notice that when you are tempted to masturbate, you are feeling lonely, bored, tired, angry, stressed, or sad. Self-pleasure, sexual fantasy and pornography, and other similar sexual activities do have an effect on the brain and are often used to tolerate, soothe, push aside, or escape unpleasant feelings. When someone uses masturbation and/or pornography as a way to escape from emotion, they can be depriving themselves of the kind of help, support, and God-centered genuine answers they truly need to tackle the real issue they may not want to face.

Conclusion

"Honor God with your body" (1 Corinthians 6:20). Amen!

EXERCISE

Take some time to journal your answers to the questions below. Then find someone you trust with whom to share your answers.

1. What have your beliefs been about masturbation before reading this chapter? Were there any things in the chapter that caused you to consider or change those beliefs?
2. What are some of the costs of engaging in pornography that you can see either in your own life or in the lives of those around you?
3. What old pathways would you like to reprogram in your brain?
4. What new ways of thinking or activities might help create a new groove of righteousness in your brain?

CHAPTER 11

THE BODY IS NOT MADE
FOR SEXUAL IMMORALITY

The Body Is for the Lord

"I have been crucified with Christ and I no longer live, but Christ lives in me. The life I now live in the body, I live by faith in the Son of God, who loved me and gave himself for me"

GALATIANS 2:20

So far in our discussion, we've thought deeply about the marvelous way God created our bodies. We've looked at the benefits of sexual purity, and seen the immense drawbacks of any sexual behavior that falls short of God's glory. But a few questions still beg to be asked. Are you absolutely convinced that sexual immorality *always* takes you outside of God's created purpose? Are you ready to do whatever it takes to live a pure life knowing that you are created for something so much greater? The Bible makes this clear. "We are his workmanship, created in Christ Jesus to do good works" (Ephesians 2:10). Our bodies are amazing and they are the workmanship of the Master Creator. Our individual physical body is the dwelling place of God. Stop. Think about that. What an absolutely amazing claim. My body is the dwelling place of the Creator of the world and the Lord of the Universe (1 Corinthians 6:18).

The work of the Holy Spirit is to sculpt us into the image of Christ. "And we all, who with unveiled faces contemplate the Lord's glory, are being transformed into his image with ever-increasing glory, which comes from the Lord, who is *the Spirit*" (2 Corinthians 3:18, emphasis added). Through our obedience to Him, God through Jesus and His Holy Spirit does this amazing work of transforming us. "The body is for the Lord" (1 Corinthians 6:13). What a powerful statement. Our body is for God. The life of Jesus is to be "manifested in our bodies" (2 Corinthians 4:9). This is a major part of the transformation of our bodies; how we use them and how we live in them. Matthew Anderson, in *Earthen Vessels,* reminds us that the God of the universe now lives in our hearts and in *our limbs.* That is such an inspiring thought. He dwells in me and can therefore transform my body and transform the habits of my body.

As you read the passages in the rest of this chapter, please keep these thoughts in mind. He loved us and sacrificed His body for us so that we would live in our bodies for Him. "The life that I now live in the body I live by faith in the Son of God who loved me and gave himself for me." Our motivation for fleeing sexual immorality comes from these amazing promises. But to solidify our convictions, we need a deeper discussion of the whole idea of sexual immorality. Why are our bodies not intended for immorality? What happens when we push past our created purpose and continue to act out sexually? Let's examine these questions.

A caveat to our readers: How this chapter could be misused: As a hammer to get someone to stop having sex; as a *scared straight* tactic to keep someone from doing something wrong sexually; to tell someone graphic details so that the very thought of having sex never enters their mind; to make someone, or even yourself, feel disgusted about the sex they just had with someone so they never do it again. Please carefully read this chapter and remember to use the material herein with wisdom and gentleness. One purpose of sharing these passages is to emphasize the importance of using the body that God gave you to bring Him glory and honor. Another purpose of this chapter is to have a blunt conversation about the very real reason God says the body is not meant for sexual immorality. However, for those of you who may already have a challenging time feeling forgiven for sexual sins you have committed in your past, consider how you may want to approach this chapter. There may be a better time and place for you to read this or you may want to read it along with someone whose spiritual guidance you trust and who can help you have a healthy response to what is shared here. Consume these words with care and wisdom.

"Food for the stomach and the stomach for food, and God will destroy them both. The body, however, is not meant/made/intended for sexual immorality but for the Lord, and the Lord for the body."

1 CORINTHIANS 6:13, VARIOUS VERSIONS ADDED

What exactly does it mean that the body is not made for sexual immorality? In a recent survey, 70-80 percent of young men and women who identify as Christians reported that they had had premarital vaginal or oral sex.[1] How could this be? It seems that many religious young men and women think oral sex is not sexual immorality and that most do not refrain from having intercourse before marriage. And how does a disciple of Jesus forge a different path?

Paul uses a clear analogy to make a strong statement here about the sexual life of someone who follows Jesus. He tells us that God made the body and that God made food. God made the body to need food. God made food to be used by the body. Both the food and the stomach can be

---

[1]   Rosenbaum, J. E., & Weathersbee, B. (2013). True love waits: Do Southern Baptists? Premarital sexual behavior among newly married Southern Baptist Sunday School students. Journal of Religion and Health, 52(1), 263-275. doi:10.1007/s10943-010-9445-5

destroyed by God. Paul here is emphasizing that God is Lord over both food and the body, and that the body and food are made for each other. However, Paul then emphasizes that although the body is made for food, the body is *not* made for sexual immorality. It is not supposed to be used for sexual immorality. God never intended the body be involved with sexual immorality. Therefore, the body is not *made* for prostitution. It is not *made* for pornography and masturbation (see chapter eleven for more on this). It is not *made* for adultery. It is not *made* for homosexual acts. It is not *made* for premarital sex. The body was not made by God for any of these acts. But why?

> "Flee from sexual immorality. All other sins a person commits are outside the body, but whoever sins sexually, sins against their own body."
>
> 1 CORINTHIANS 6:18

It is so important that we understand one of the reasons God says, "Flee." The word here is *pheugo* in the Greek, meaning *shun, escape.* Joseph ran when Pharaoh's wife asked him to have sex with her (Genesis 49:12). Why? Well, we know that we are actually called to flee from any type of sin (1 Corinthians 10:14, 1 Timothy 6:11, 2 Timothy 2:22). Yet Paul, in 1 Corinthians 6:18, says that sexual sin has a greater impact on the body.

What are some of the results of having sex before you are married? What impact does having sex with someone else other than your spouse have when you are married? What happens to our body and brain when we have sex before marriage, with someone other than our spouse, or someone of the same sex? What happens to our bodies when we become involved in sexually immoral things like pornography, strip clubs or cybersex? What impact does masturbation have on our body, our psyche, and the wiring of our brain?

Men and women ask these questions regularly in workshops and counseling appointments. People wonder if the things they have done, or are doing, or things that have been done to them, have messed up their body, soul, or spirit in some way. In all reality, this is a complex question to answer because the brain, the emotions, the body, the spirit, and the psyche are influenced by and influence each other in rather complicated ways. Let's begin by examining some of the literal physical manifestations on the body.

The Physiological Effects of Sexual Abuse

Being a victim of sexual trauma is obviously not a choice anyone makes. Therefore, why would we include addressing the physiological effects of sexual abuse in this chapter? We share the information here because of the number of people concerned about how their bodies have been affected by sexual trauma. Often these questions have come up in the context of someone getting help with the very real ways individuals experience their bodies after a violation.

There are bodily, psychological, spiritual, and emotional tolls for those who experience sexual violations of any kind. Some of this is covered in chapter six, *Sexual Abuse*. However, for this section, let's consider the physiological effects of sexual abuse. Once again, for those of you reading here, if this is your background, make sure you have support before reading this passage. If reading this becomes difficult, you may want to pause and breathe, or even wait until you are with a trusted friend before you read on.

When someone is sexually assaulted, there can be physical consequences, such as torn tissues, bruising, and blood loss. The sexual assault could also result in pregnancy in male to female assault. For women, sexual abuse can also lead to issues with their menstrual cycle or problems with fertility. Because sexual abuse also causes high levels of stress, a person may experience chronic fatigue, shortness of breath, muscle tension, involuntary and random moments of shaking and challenges with eating and sleeping. The immediate and long-term responses to sexual assault or molestation can range anywhere from hypervigilance and avoidance of sex to sexual risk-taking and promiscuity. Each of these responses can cause physiological harm, such as the biological effects of stress on the body from constant vigilance, including high adrenaline and high cortisol levels, and the possible increased chance of STDs and pelvic floor trauma.

There can also be some longer-term physical and sexual results from sexual abuse or assault. I (Jennifer) have worked with married men who were experiencing sexual problems in their marital sexual relationship. Men who experienced penetrative or forced penetration sexual violations during childhood and adolescence (rape and molestation) had a higher rate of erectile dysfunction.[2] Women who experienced a high rate of negative sexual events (see the list in chapters four and six, *The Development of the Sexual Self* and *Sexual Abuse*) had higher rates of problems in sexual functioning including sexual pain, difficulties reaching orgasm, and low sexual desire. For both men and women, those who have experienced sexual abuse or rape have a higher incidence of sexual problems, such as pelvic floor pain and arousal problems.

For further understanding of the physiological consequences of all forms of abuse, including sexual trauma, look up the Ted Talk by Nadine Burke Harris on "How Childhood Trauma Affects Health Across a Lifetime."

If you have experienced or are experiencing any of these physiological challenges, you may need to seek professional care. It is also important to remember that God is the Great Healer. "I am the Lord who heals you" (Exodus 15:26). At times, shame and embarrassment can keep us from seeking out medical or spiritual help, but it is at these times that reaching out to God and to compassionate others can put us on the road to true healing.

---

[2]   Konzen, J. (2014). The EIS model: A mixed methods research study of a multidisciplinary sex therapy treatment. (Doctoral Dissertation). Available from ProQuest Dissertations and Theses database. (UMI No. 11722)

The Body and Premarital and Extramarital Sex

A common thought in the secular world is that there are health benefits to having an active sex life, especially one that is not restricted by the religious or moral belief that sex should only occur in marriage. One Internet author contends that "having sex before marriage ... can bolster happiness and lead to a longer life, and it 'releases stress, boosts immunities, helps you sleep, and is heart-healthy.'" One might think this is just indicative of the thinking in the secular world, but polls of Christians reveal similar viewpoints. Obviously, the teaching in the Scriptures that the body is not made for sexual immorality is contrary to this kind of thinking. What is a disciple of Jesus supposed to believe?

To answer this, we need to look at some of the obvious effects of sex outside of marriage. (Note that these can occur during marriage as well.) Most teenagers who have watched the puberty film at school know that STDs (like chlamydia, HIV, herpes, etc.) can result from sex, especially if sex is unprotected. Statistics show that the rate of contraction of STDs is much higher for those involved in premarital and extramarital sex. Pregnancy can also be an obvious physiological result.

For many, however, the results of sex outside of marriage are not as obviously physical. For instance, one research study found that when young women have sex earlier than their peers, they have higher rates of depression, especially when those relationships break up.[3] Premarital sex and sex outside of marriage can also create certain sexual expectations. You might come to expect sex to always have that level of thrill (the thrill of the forbidden or the new, or the thrill of the chase).

When you get married, you might experience dissatisfaction with marital sex, because it is not accompanied with that same level of physical arousal and sexual excitement you experienced from the danger or illicitness of your sexual experiences before marriage. Also, if sex is pleasurable with a premarital partner, you may compare sex with your

---

[3]   Meier, A. (2007). Adolescent first sex and subsequent mental health. American Journal of Sociology, 112/6, 1-28.

spouse to previous partners, even if you never say this out loud. This is especially true if sex in your marriage is not going well, or if you are having sexual functioning problems you did not have with previous partners, or even if your partner doesn't seem as "romantic." Think how guilty you might feel about these kinds of things and how difficult it would be to share them with your spouse. These comparisons especially come out when the marriage is in distress, even when they are not openly stated. Remember, as a single person you are laying the groundwork for how you will view and physiologically experience sexuality in marriage.

There has also been some interesting research specific to having affairs in marriage (extramarital sex). A research study in 2012 found that men are more likely to die during sexual intercourse when they are having an extramarital sexual relationship.[4] These researchers found that being unfaithful was a risk factor for major adverse cardiovascular events. Wow!

What the Scriptures teach is that sex creates a one-flesh bond between two people. "That is why a man leaves his father and mother and is united to his wife, and they become one flesh" (Genesis 2:24). And when you sleep with anyone before or outside of marriage, even someone you pay, your flesh is becoming one with theirs. "Do you not know that he who unites himself with a prostitute is one with her in body? For it is said, 'The two will become one flesh'" (1 Corinthians 6:16). This is a little hard to believe at face value. Most people will say that when they have sex with a paid sex worker, it is not any kind of an emotional bond and there is no lasting physical connection. But the Scriptures say otherwise. God says otherwise. And we, therefore, believe that this is physiologically true in a way that, although hard to grasp, is nevertheless accurate.

The woman stalking Tom Cruise in the movie *Vanilla Sky* said it very well: "Don't you know that when you sleep with someone, your body

---

4   Fisher, A. D., Bandini, E., Corona, G., Monami, M., Cameron Smith, M., Melani, C., Balzi, D., Forti, G., Mannucci, E. and Maggi, M. (2012). Stable extramarital affairs are breaking the heart. International Journal of Andrology, 35, 11–17. doi:10.1111/j.1365- 2605.2011.01176.x

makes a promise whether you do or not?" Below, we will explore this further.

The Effects of Pornography and Masturbation

We have already mentioned the spiritual, emotional, and psychological effects of pornography in chapter ten, *Masturbation and Pornography*. However, we want to include here a very brief mention of other physiological effects of pornography and masturbation.

There are a number of different things that can happen when someone gets involved in compulsive masturbation and pornography. One study called "Who is screwing around here?" found that religious individuals who consumed pornography against their religious values were much more likely to engage in extramarital affairs than religious individuals who did not consume pornography.[5] Likewise, as even a single consumption of porn often creates an ever-increasing appetite making you more likely to eventually find a way to be sexually involved with real people, pornography is like a *gateway drug* that leads to sex before or outside of marriage.

Porn use before marriage can also impact how you function one day within marriage. There is a sharp rise in erectile dysfunction, delayed ejaculation, decreased sexual satisfaction, and diminished libido for men involved in pornography and compulsive masturbation.[6] Research has found that these behaviors alter the brain's motivational system and condition someone's sexual arousal to be connected to viewing Internet pornography. This is believed to be the result of Internet-pornography-induced alterations in the circuits of the brain that govern sexual desire and penile erection. This is much like the chronic and compulsive abuse

---

[5]   Huey, K. M. (2004). Who is screwing around here? The relationship between religiosity, pornography, and extramarital sex. Dissertation Abstracts International, 64, 3510.

[6]   Park, B. Y., Wilson, G., Berger, J., Christman, M., Reina, B., Bishop, F.,... Doan, A. P.(2016). Is internet pornography causing sexual dysfunctions? A review with clinical reports. Behavioral Sciences, 6(3), 17. http://doi.org/10.3390/bs6030017

of drugs or engaging in gambling. An individual can get used to pornography triggering greater arousal and faster and stronger orgasms. These alterations and wired preferences can then cause problems with your ability to one day be physically aroused by your spouse. Stopping internet pornography can reverse this, but the process can be long and difficult.

The Body, Sex, and Your Relationship with God

One research study done in 2009 found that when men are extrinsically motivated in their religious life, they are more likely to engage in extramarital sex.[7] What does that mean? Extrinsic motivation is when someone chooses to behave a certain way because of the outward rewards they receive, such as money, praise, grades/promotions, and fame/good reputation. This type of motivation rises from external circumstances. Intrinsic motivation, on the other hand, is when behavior choices are driven by more internal factors like internal satisfaction, joy, meaning, and personal values and beliefs. This study then found that men whose reasons for staying away from sex were based on external factors—what others would think or the negative consequences that could happen if they engaged in sex—were more likely to have sex outside of the marital relationship. It is therefore vital that we set our eyes on Jesus, the author and perfecter of our faith. Our motivation needs to be to please Him as Jesus did. "I always do what pleases Him" (John 16:8). For most, extrinsic motivating factors, like getting STDs or the possibility of getting someone pregnant, do not stop people from engaging in extramarital sexual relationships. Working diligently to be in awe of God, being guided by a genuine knowing of who God is, is the intrinsic motivation that protects the body from the physical consequences of extramarital sexuality.

---

[7]   DeMaris, A. (2009). Distal and Proximal Influences on the Risk of Extramarital Sex: A Prospective Study of Longer Duration Marriages. Journal of Sex Research, 46(6), 597–607.

Two Become One

There are a number of scriptures that address the body and sexuality, and especially the idea that when two people engage in sex, those two bodies become one flesh. However, God has specific direction on which bodies should be having sex together and what bodies we are not supposed to have sex with. Let's look further at these scriptures.

> "You are not your own. You were bought with a price. Therefore honor God with your bodies."
>
> 1 Corinthians 6:19-20

> "It is God's will that you should be sanctified: that you should avoid sexual immorality; that each of you should learn to control your own body in a way that is holy and honorable, not in passionate lust like the pagans, who do not know God."
>
> 1 Thessalonians 4:4-5

> "A man shall leave his father and his mother, and be joined to his wife; and they shall become one flesh."
>
> Genesis 2:24; Matt 19:5

> "Your bodies are members of Christ himself? Shall I then take the members of Christ and unite them with a prostitute? Never!...But whoever is united with the Lord is one with him in spirit...Do you not know that your bodies are temples of the Holy Spirit, who is in you, whom you have received from God? You are not your own."
>
> 1 Corinthians 6:15-18

The Corinthians believed that sexual activity was a mere bodily function like eating food. This led them to the conclusion that normal bodily functions had no abiding significance and were, therefore, of no ultimate consequence. Paul uses the words "Do you not know?" several times when he discusses sexual immorality with them to show very real and urgent concern. How can you not know this? In fact, I know you know this because everybody knows this. And this is never to happen. Ever. The use of the word "Never" shows the idea of having sex with a prostitute for a Christian is an absolute, vehement no. Therefore, sexual sin like this was *unthinkable* for the Christian. It was not an option.

If we are to follow the Bible's sexual ethic, we have to embrace the absoluteness of this passage. The only real sex in life, according to the God who created us, is the sex that happens within the covenant of marriage. All the rest is imitation. And the reality is, there are some very realistic imitations. In fact, for most people, when they eat the imitation, they would never know it wasn't real. Like the product "I Can't Believe It's Not Butter." It just tastes so good that I know it's the real thing. When people have sex outside of marriage, they often say it's great. It tasted great! It felt physically great! Their body enjoyed it. But if we believe the Bible is true, then we know, no matter how we feel emotionally, no matter what level of enjoyment our body says we are having, the only kind of sex that is genuinely physically and bodily fulfilling is that which is found in marriage between a husband and wife.

When you look at Leviticus 18, God lists all the people we are not supposed to have sex with. Having sex with these individuals is not what the body was created to do: your mother, your father's wife (stepmom), your sister, your father's daughter (whether she was born in the same home or elsewhere), your son's daughter (granddaughter), your daughter's daughter (granddaughter), your father's wife's daughter (stepsister), your father's sister (your aunt), your mother's sister (your aunt), your father's brother's wife (your aunt by marriage), your daughter-in-law, your brother's wife (your sister-in-law), a woman and her daughter, a woman and her son's daughter or her daughter's daughter (a woman and her granddaughter), and your wife's sister (your sister-in-law).

OK. We get the picture. Or maybe we don't. Maybe that is why God has to go into such extremely specific detail. He says, "No one is to approach any close relative to have sexual relations," and then He takes eleven more verses to make sure we understand what He means. Then the list in Deuteronomy 18 adds three more individuals we are not to have sex with. Your neighbor's wife, another man (if you are a man), or an animal.

Over and over He says having sex with any of these is dishonorable. When we are sexually immoral, we dishonor our own bodies, we dishonor other people and their bodies, and we dishonor (even if you aren't married yet) the one place where sex is supposed to happen—in the marriage bed. And this scripture shows how this is true whether someone feels that way emotionally or not. God says that those who do these things defile or contaminate themselves. God is not asking us to go about putting scarlet letters on those who commit sexual sin. He is not calling us to go and shout "defiled" to anyone who has sex before they are married. He is not calling us to treat someone who commits adultery as defiled. He does not want us walking around saying to ourselves "I am defiled" (we will expand on this more in chapter twelve, *Save Yourself*). However, He is clearly stating that sex isn't supposed to be done this way with any body other than the body we are married to. We were literally not created to do this. The body is not made for sexual immorality and it does not show honor to the body that God made when we do.

God's Authority

It is vital that we remember that *because we are the very dwelling place of the Holy Spirit, our bodies are not our own to do with as we please.* We do not have the authority to live in our body according to our own desires. Anderson in *Earthen Vessels* reminds us that although our current culture screams that freedom gives us the absolute right to do whatever we want as long as we do not "harm" others, Scripture teaches us otherwise. Our bodies are God's instruments, as if God were doing His very work through us (Ephesians 2:10). As followers of Jesus, we are called to submit our body to the authority of God and this is a good thing because the God who made our body knows what is best for that body.

Remember the reader's caveat at the beginning of this chapter? Please do not use these scriptures to condemn yourself or to condemn those who have committed sexual sins. Let God decide what to do with that. Let Jesus be the decision maker on that one (John 8:11). He does a pretty good job of being that decision maker in this passage in John 8. Imitate Him and use these teachings and scriptures to build a healthy, biblical understanding of the heart of God and the truth of His Word. He adores us. We are His. And He gave us our body so that we might use it in a way to honor Him and so that we would enjoy life to the full. So honor God with your body and flee from sexual immorality. Then do lots of other great things with your body like serve the poor, clean someone's toilet, cook a meal for someone, or fix someone's car, and then enjoy holy, passionate sex when you're married!

Singlehood And Sex

CHAPTER 12

SAVE YOURSELF

Purity rings. Promises to wait. Saving sex for marriage. Not giving away your virginity. Waiting to give it to your wife, your husband. There are so many different ways to describe the decision to save yourself, to choose to refrain from having sex until you are married. I (Jennifer) received a text from my daughter while she was serving in an orphanage in Africa. These were her exact words: "Hey, can you answer this question for me biblically? Why should you save sex for marriage? And why can't it be experienced before instead of waiting 'til after?:) Thanks, you're the best." I had this momentary concern about just what she was doing in that faraway country, but we ended up having a digital conversation laughing about how these questions were for some girls she was reaching out to. I loved that she asked, and I loved that this was one way she was sharing her faith. What is funny is that I had to do some of my own study to make sure I gave her some solid answers.

So does the Bible really teach that sex should occur only in marriage and that premarital sex is not in God's plan? This is a valid question. And some of the answers people give to say there is nothing wrong with premarital sex sound pretty good. They say that sex is an expression of love and God is a god of love. Therefore, surely God would not disapprove as long as we love, are not harming anyone, and we are committed to each other. There are, in fact, books written that claim these very things.[1] If someone asked you whether sex before marriage is wrong, you might be tempted to give the answer, "Of course." If you have asked someone this question, you may have gotten an angry or trite answer. It is important to take some time to examine what the Bible does say about premarital sex. However, this can be challenging because the words *premarital sex* are not found in the Bible. The Bible talks about sex before marriage, and the Bible talks about sexual acts that occur outside of marriage. However, the specific term *premarital sex*, though a common term today, is not found in Scripture. In the following section, you will find some of the Scriptures (and a few others) that we used to answer Jacqueline that day in Africa all the way from San Diego.

Before going through the Scriptures below to look at what the Bible says about premarital sex, we want to address those who have already engaged in premarital or extramarital sex. It is very important to remember that anyone who chooses to do God's will, even if they have engaged in sex before marriage, can be pure in God's eyes and pursue a lifestyle of purity.

> "Remember, O Lord, your great mercy and love ... Remember not the sins of my youth or my rebellious ways; according to your love remember me, for you are good, O Lord."
>
> PSALMS 25:6-7

I (Tim) did not practice sexual self-control until shortly before the day I made Jesus Lord at age twenty-seven. I had to do a lot of confessing to spiritual men I trusted before that day. When we turn to Jesus and come into the light, confess our sins (James 5:16), and then are washed in His blood at baptism (1 Pet 3:21, Acts 22:16), we need to remember that His blood cleanses us (1 John 1:7) and that we are once again made pure, cleansed from all unrighteousness (1 John 1:10). My wife was a virgin

---

[1]   McCleneghan, B. (2016). Good Christian Sex: Why chastity isn't the only option – and other things the bible says about sex. HarperOne.

when we got married. What a gift to me. What she believed, and I knew was true because the Bible says it, was that in God's eyes, I also was pure at our wedding. Thank you, God, for the blood of your Son. So if this describes you, if you have repented of a sexual past that happened before Christ or as a Christian, sex that was not according to the Scriptures, remember, as a repentant, baptized, grateful disciple of Jesus, you are made pure; He remembers you according to His love. And now, how does God want you to conduct your life in the area of sexuality if you are not yet married?

What Scripture Says

Before you read on, we want to emphasize that the Scriptures below are to help each of us understand the doctrinally correct view of sex before marriage. However, please remember these scriptures are not to be used in any manner that is not consistent with the heart of God. Using them as a hammer, either on yourself or on others, would not be handling the Scriptures correctly. Look to the attitude, heart, and conviction of Jesus in John 8 to get a perfect illustration of how to handle God's Word with grace and truth.

There are quite a number of Scriptures in the Old Testament about sexual immorality, and, as we will see, all of these can apply to premarital sex. However, the most blunt is found in Deuteronomy. Here, God lays out a clear consequence of premarital sex. "If a man happens to meet in a town a virgin pledged to be married and he sleeps with her, you shall take both of them to the gate of that town and stone them to death" (Deuteronomy 22:23-24). In one concise statement, God made it very clear His stance on premarital sex.

Then we see God *live on stage* in John 8:1-11. A woman caught in adultery and she is brought to Jesus as they prepare to stone her. This is where we continue to see the heart of God. Let's look at the whole passage. "The teachers of the law and the Pharisees brought in a woman caught in adultery. They made her stand before the group and said to

Jesus, 'Teacher, this woman was caught in the act of adultery. In the Law Moses commanded us to stone such women. Now what do you say?' " (John 8:3-6)

Here we see the teachers of the law telling the Creator of that law what it says. And then they try to catch Him out. "What do you say?" And what *does* He say? "Let any one of you who is without sin be the first to throw a stone at her" (v. 7). When they drop their stones and leave, God in the flesh tells the woman, "Neither do I condemn you. Go now and leave your life of sin" (v.11).

So God tells us bluntly that we are not to engage in premarital or extramarital sex and that there are consequences when we do. And then He takes the punishment and provides the cleansing if we do engage in sexual immorality before or during marriage. As with the woman caught in adultery, Jesus then adds directly and pointedly, "Go now and leave your life of sin." We can imitate Him and be clear on what is wrong and be clear on His grace and mercy *at the same time*, letting His grace and mercy continually move us into repentance.

In the New Testament, the most common Scripture used to explain how God views sex outside of marriage is Hebrews 13:4. "Marriage should be honored by all, and the marriage bed kept pure, for God will judge the adulterer and all the sexually immoral." It helps to look at several reliable translations to get a full sense of the meaning of these words. One of these is the New Living Translation: "Give honor to marriage, and remain faithful to one another in marriage. God will surely judge people who are immoral and those who commit adultery." Another is the Holman Christian Standard which says, "Marriage must be respected by all, and the marriage bed kept undefiled, because God will judge immoral people and adulterers."

These translations make it clear that adultery, as spoken of in many other Scriptures as well, is clearly outside of God's plan. What is interesting about this Scripture in Hebrews is that sexual immorality here is clearly defined as something other than adultery. "God will judge the adulterer and all the sexually immoral." The meaning in the Greek for the word here is any sex outside of the marriage relationship other than adultery. It would be like saying "adultery and any other sex that happens but is not between two married people" or "sex with someone other than your spouse and everything else sexual." That is how one defiles the marriage bed—not just during extramarital sex (adultery), but at any other time that sex is occurring when someone is not in a marital relationship.

Jesus defines this even clearer. If someone even thinks about another with lust in their heart or mind, they are committing adultery. "I tell you that anyone who looks at a woman lustfully has already committed adultery with her in his heart" (Matthew 5:28). You don't even have to be married to commit adultery. You can be a single individual looking at any man or woman in a sexual way. These Scriptures fit within the entire sexual ethic as found in the Scriptures. Paul says in 1 Corinthians 6:16 that when someone has sex with a prostitute, they become one flesh. And why is that so seriously wrong? Because it defies the very purpose God intended for sex. God tells us in Genesis 2:24 that when a man leaves his parents and bonds with his wife, the "two become one flesh." That one flesh relationship happens in the marital relationship. Paul is telling the disciples in Corinth that when they sleep with a prostitute, they take the *one flesh* bonding that is meant for the sexual relationship in marriage and have it with someone they are not married to, a prostitute. Sex unites and joins two bodies (1 Corinthians 6:16-17) whether you care about that person or not; whether you paid for sex or you love someone; whether you are single or married. God intended that bonding, that one flesh unity, for the marital sexual relationship. And any sex that occurs outside of that is the defiling spoken about in Hebrews 13:4.

It is also important to note what is defiled in this Scripture. It is the marriage bed that is defiled, not the person committing the act. We can often use this Scripture to say that someone is defiled if they commit sexual sin. Many have said they feel defiled. But we want to point out that though there is no question that sin messes up our lives, the point God is making here is not "You are defiled!" But having sex outside of marriage defiles the beauty of sex as it was created by God. We know that any sin we commit can separate us from God and that we are all in desperate need of the continually cleansing blood of Jesus. Sexual sin, however, will often lead to people feeling like *they* are defiled and too dirty for God to save. This is not the focus of this Scripture. God is saying here that the marriage bed is a place of beauty and purity and that He wants us to thoroughly enjoy that bed as He created it to be. He wants us to stay away from everything both before and during marriage that could take away from that beauty. Praise God that He can restore beauty (Isaiah 61:3) even when we do things that allow contamination. And praise God that He gives us direction how to stay away from all that contaminates.

Again, in 1 Corinthians 7:2, Paul makes this point that sex is for marriage even more clear as he tells men and women that "because of sexual immorality, each man should have his own wife, and each woman should have her own husband" (HCSB). He tells the unmarried, "If they cannot control themselves, they should marry, for it is better to marry than to burn with passion" (1 Corinthians 7:9). Because Paul wants to be very sure we get this message, after emphasizing that he thinks it is better to remain unmarried, he says again, "If anyone is worried that he might not be acting honorably toward the virgin he is engaged to, and if his passions are too strong and he feels he ought to marry, he should do as he wants. He is not sinning. They should get married" (1 Corinthians 7:36).

Other translations can help further our understanding. "If a man thinks that he's treating his fiancée improperly" (New Living Translation) and "if anyone thinks that he is not behaving properly toward his betrothed" (English Standard Version). So, clearly, if you are tempted to be sexually immoral (have sex outside of marriage), if you burn for sex and feel you cannot control that burn, get direction from godly advisers about whether you should get married. If you are possibly *acting improperly* or *not honorably* with someone you are engaged to, get direction and consider moving up the wedding date. With those advisers, explore if the burn comes from any unhealthy desire for sex, if there has been pressure from a partner to have sex, or if the desire to engage sexually comes from a desire to feel loved. These may be signs that marriage may not be the best plan. Explore where the burn is from, and consider if pursuing marriage is God's direction for you.

And then remember, the place to act on that burn, the place to *act properly* sexually, the place to engage in the sexual relationship, is only after you get married. "May you ever be intoxicated with her love" (Proverbs 5:19). God intends sex to be intoxicating, but the place He wants that intoxication to happen is within the married relationship. Of course this doesn't mean that you want to rush into a marriage just in order not to be sexually immoral or so that you can have sex. However, it does emphasize where God intends sex to happen.

So, if you are wondering if the Bible teaches that sex is only meant for marriage, and if premarital sex is outside of His plan, these Scriptures show us an unequivocal yes and yes.

Your Blueprint

When a building is constructed, architects and construction workers use a blueprint. When we decide to follow Jesus, He says we need to sit down and estimate the cost before we build a building (Luke 14:28). When we go into a committed dating relationship or an engaged relationship, it is important to look and see if our blueprint is a good one. Is this the building you want? Look at your blueprint when it comes to sexuality. Is it based on models from the world, from the movies, from magazines? Male and female health magazines, romance novels, chick flicks, and popular TV shows tell us what love is supposed to look like. Using popular movies and shows, Satan has made sexual immorality look very enticing. In the movie *Titanic*, there is a classic scene in a carriage that is full of emotion, attraction, and highly charged intimacy. It's an incredibly romantic, erotic scene. And they are not married. Yet most every person who has watched that scene remembers it. Those scenes not only affect our expectation of the sexual relationship, but they may also offer a blueprint of what is acceptable to do intimately before marriage. Is that the blueprint you have? Are you aware of your blueprint and of how much that blueprint could be influencing you? Our culture demeans marital sex and instead celebrates immoral sex. Are you aware of the messages and the blueprint that is underneath those messages?

We can gain more insight by examining the messages the world gives about those who wait to have sex until marriage. For instance, we can examine why the typical person hasn't had sex. One study done in the 90s found that the primary reason conservative religious college students had not yet had sex was that they had not been in a relationship long enough or hadn't fallen in love. They were also concerned with AIDS and pregnancy. Religious beliefs were *seventh* on the list for women and *ninth* for men. In a secular study[2] done more recently, the reason why people chose to have sex were physical ("the person had beautiful eyes," "a desirable body," or was "too attractive to resist"); emotional (wanting to "communicate on a deeper level," "lift my partner's spirits"); to attain a goal (to retaliate on a cheating partner, "be popular," or "because of a bet"); or to combat insecurity ("my duty," "my self-esteem").

It can be helpful to take a good look at some of the thinking that might be influencing your own. Don't just glance quickly. Look closely and genuinely. If you don't look honestly, these very things can pull you toward engaging sexually sooner than your values and love for God would direct you. Deepen your roots in God's Word so that you can look to the God who created you when you make the choice of how to live sexually.

Dating Couples

"How far should we go?" This is a common question that dating couples ask. You may be asking, "We want to stay pure, so how far is too far?" In today's world, the definition of what is considered sex does not always match that within Scripture. When a world leader who has had oral sex says, "I did not have sexual relations with that woman," and when it is

---

2   Meston, C., & Buss, D. (2007). Why humans have sex. Archives of Sexual Behavior,36(4), 477-507.

common for young couples to say that they are refraining from sex but are still giving each other orgasms, it can be confusing trying to figure out where the line of "too far" lies. Many couples will use worldly guides that are not based on Scriptures to decide these lines. "Well, at least we haven't had intercourse," as if intercourse is the sum total of sex. This is why it is so freeing to have the Scriptures as a guide.

"Among you there must not be even a hint of sexual immorality... because these are improper for God's holy people" (Ephesians 5:3). The Greek word here for *hint* literally means *let it not be named*. Let it not even be mentioned. Don't even come close enough to talk to it. Just using this one scripture, it is clear that giving someone oral sex or bringing them to orgasm is definitely in the naming or hint category. In fact, it is quite a bit beyond naming and mentioning. A hint might be more like making a sexual innuendo, or brushing across or pressing up against the breast, buttocks, or penis, or the throbbing and tingling that continues when we dwell on lustful thoughts and feelings. We learned earlier that the initial physiological reaction of blood flow that comes instantaneously when someone thinks a sexual thought or sees something sexual is the God-created bodily reaction to sexual stimuli. What we do with it after we notice that reaction is when we enter the realm of choice; either opening ourselves up to and indulging that hint or choosing the path of purity even when we are in an intimate relationship with another. There is an almost laughable place where this *hint*, or naming, is spelled out, even in the secular world. In the school district that our children attend, the students are required to sign a student handbook. Many of them have never read it. Yet hidden in its pages are these words: "Public Display of Affection: In an effort to promote behavior which establishes a friendly atmosphere without causing others to feel embarrassment or discomfort, unacceptable are: prolonged or heavy kissing; fondling/inappropriate sexual contact; excessive body contact."

This requirement might turn out to be a good starting place for most of us when it comes to deciding what kind of physical behavior we will not engage in while we are dating or engaged. At this point, it could be helpful to backtrack from there and figure out what kind of situations make it "too easy" to indulge in these kinds of choices.

The goal, according to the apostle Paul in Ephesians 5:3, is to only engage in what is proper. With this Scripture in mind, it is clear that purposefully pursuing any action that causes sexual arousal would be beyond what is proper in a premarital relationship. Also, proper conduct may depend on the level of commitment in the relationship. A couple who is early in their dating relationship versus a couple on the eve of marrying might have different definitions of what would be considered proper at that point in their relationship. We somewhat get an indication of that when Timothy is told by Paul to treat the younger women as sisters (1 Timothy 5:2) with absolute purity. And then, as we saw in Corinthians, Paul tells men that if they are engaged, there are things they might be doing that are improper (1 Corinthians 7:36). There is some kind of progression from absolute purity toward conduct that is not honorable. They are behaving in some way that is not proper or honorable to those *unpresentable parts* that are mentioned in 1 Corinthians 12:23.

So for a couple in an exclusive relationship, what would *proper* include? Is petting and touching the genitals too far? Is placing a finger in her vagina too far? Is stroking his penis too far? Is French kissing too far? Is grasping the buttocks too far? Is caressing the stomach too far? Rather, the more appropriate question might be: Is petting or genital touch a hint? We would say absolutely. What about French kissing, touching the buttocks, or caressing the stomach? Lauren Winner makes a suggestion in *Real Sex*. She talks about the input a ministry leader gave her and her fiancée. "Don't do anything sexual you wouldn't be comfortable doing on the steps of the rotunda," the rotunda being a domed gazebo at the center of the campus. In *Soul Virgins*, Douglas Rosenau and Michael Wilson talk about committed couples (by this they mean engaged) enjoying intimate touch that does not go beyond the bikini zone. Though this can be a helpful guideline, what is covered by a bikini is continually shifting as bikinis now include G-strings with full buttocks showing. Also, a bikini guideline does not address touching of the male body and a pursuit of purity would address not only a "bikini" area but any other intimate touches that may be important to consider.

Our recommendation is that *proper* definitely includes this combination of input: Take into consideration what you'd feel is appropriate if you were somewhere other people might show up and use this as your physical guideline. However you decide, an important issue to contemplate is not the exact amount of touching that should happen, but what you are aiming for in your relationship.

If you are aiming for how often you can receive that physical jolt and sexual buzz, your relationship may already be well beyond the hint. If you are pressing the boundaries, seeing how close you can get to the edge, you may want to take a good look at your convictions and your relationship with God.

Looking at this from a view of honoring God, your aim can be instead to build one another up. Think of Ephesians 4:29, "Do not let any unwholesome talk come out of your mouths, but only what is helpful for building others up according to their needs, that it may benefit those who listen." Apply this to the choices you make to what kind of touch to engage in in your relationship. "Do not let any unwholesome touch come from your hands, but only the kind of touch that is helpful for building up your boyfriend/girlfriend according to their needs, that it may benefit them when you touch them." Benefit one another and build each other up in how you touch. Honor the other in a way that helps guard the decision you have each made to wait for sexual touch until marriage.

Engaged Couples

Preparing for marriage, and preparing for an enjoyable, God honoring sexual relationship, can be and should be filled with fun and excitement. For those in committed, engaged relationships, light touches to the neck and stomach may be enjoyable and a good progress toward marriage. However, if approaching that kind of intimate touch leads to outcomes that make remaining pure both in thought and action difficult, having a good conversation about that both together and with those you trust can help a couple decide what is best for them. If you engage in something where you find yourself sexually aroused (a throbbing vagina or erect penis), if it becomes difficult to keep your thoughts from picturing having sex together, if you find yourself more drawn to masturbation, these may be indications that perhaps your boundaries could use a reassessment. This isn't about feeling guilt over sexual attraction. Sexual feelings can happen when someone you love and are attracted to takes your hand and bites your knuckle. However, without being overcome with guilt, frustration, or resentment, take a genuine look and have a healthy conversation.

Obviously, 1 Corinthians 7:36 could suggest that if you are having a hard time staying inside proper intimacy, you either move up the wedding date or you pull back on what you're doing intimately However, if you find yourself habitually caught in a snare of sexual immorality (continually seeking sexual gratification), then it may be time to consider a journey of recovering godly sexual integrity—always remembering that God's mercy and compassion is a safety net that allows you to be fully involved in the genuine, deep work of maintaining purity, even within a committed relationship.

Some couples make a decision to save even kissing for the wedding. That was the decision we made. We had seen so much immorality, even within the singles ministry we led, and we had no desire to go down that road. So when I (Tim) asked Jennifer to be my girlfriend, I let her know I was not planning on kissing. Our first kiss was at our wedding. And we did a lot of kissing after that (see the smile). Now mind you, because of our longstanding friendship, both our dating relationship and our engagement were each a little over two months (four-and-a-half months total). So we don't share this as an expectation for everyone. We share it as our experience, which may not be what you need.

In fact, there are some couples who not only decide not to kiss, but they also have almost no physical contact, even finding some discomfort in holding hands. For some, this lack of appropriate intimate touch may actually lead to problems once married. For them, finding pure ways to engage in healthy enjoyment of a godly physical relationship may be important and needed. Some of my (Jennifer's) favorite memories during our dating and engagement are of how Tim would hold my hand. His thumb would slide over my fingers with a gentle caressing motion. It was definitely sensual and enjoyable. In your pursuit of purity as an engaged couple, enjoying appropriate physical touch is good and godly. Figuring out what that means for your relationship is usually a matter of prayer, laughter, godly direction, and honest conversation.

EXERCISES

Sexual Choices Exercise:
Godly Intimacy for Committed Couples

If you are in a committed relationship, use the following questions with the accompanying Scriptures to explore together what you want to include in your physical intimacy while dating/engaged. Though the questions mention a fiancée, they can also be applied to committed dating couples.

What's Allowed:
Five Questions to Guide Your Sexual Choices Before Marriage.

1. Is it prohibited by Scripture (i.e., lust, sexual immorality, a hint: Matthew 5:28, Galatians 5:19-21, Ephesians 5:3)?
2. Is it beneficial and constructive (1 Corinthians 10:23-24)? Does it benefit and build up your relationship, and are you seeking your fiancée's good?
3. Does it lead to picturing sex with your fiancée or anyone else (fantasizing — Hebrews 13:4, Matthew 5:28)?
4. What is the fruit (Matthew 7:16-20)? When you put it into

practice, does it create connection between you? Does it lead to anything detrimental or to a lack of proper intimacy (1 Corinthians 7:36)?

5. Does it violate your or your fiancée's conscience (Romans 14:5, 1 Corinthians 8:7-13)?

CHAPTER 13

QUESTIONS SINGLES, TEENS, AND STUDENTS HAVE ABOUT SEX

When you saw the title of this book, what did you think? Often when those who are not married hear about a class for them on sexuality, they think, "Great, another lesson on purity." However, some of you might have seen the title and felt, "Finally, it's about time somebody talked about this." Others of you might feel like avoiding the whole topic because all it leads to is frustration, guilt, and confusion.

When we have run workshops, participants let us know what they were needing, and that has always helped guide what we cover. If someone were to ask you about what kinds of challenges you are facing in the area of sexuality, what would you answer? If you were asked about what fears, concerns, or questions you have about sex, what would you say? Below is a list of questions we have received from teens, campus students, and singles. They are word for word what they asked and we will attempt to answer them.

Why can't I touch my body if I am not arousing others? It is only my body anyways. If my mind is just blank, and I'm not thinking of any person, is masturbation a sin?

This is such a valid question. Go ahead and read chapter one, *What Does the Bible Say About Sex*, chapter ten, *Masturbation and Pornography*, and chapter five on *Body Image*. Bottom line, there is no scripture that says you can't touch your body. There also are no scriptures that directly say you cannot arouse yourself. Many times, the Bible doesn't have specific direction to what is God's will for a specific question (something like: "Should I buy that car?") In those cases, we have to look at scriptural principles or how scriptures might tie together.

Here are some verses that address some aspect of this question:

1. "Do not stir up (arouse, NIV) or awaken love until *the appropriate time*" (Song of Songs 2:7, 3:5, 8:4, HCSB);
2. Scriptures that make it clear that sex is for marriage (see chapter twelve on *Save Yourself*);
3. "Anyone who looks at a woman lustfully has already committed adultery with her in his heart" (Matthew 5:28).

This last Scripture makes it clear that looking with feelings of lust is a sin. Most individuals will admit that they fantasize (looking at a picture in their mind) when they masturbate. Being aroused or stirred up does have an *appropriate time*, and God's plan for that appropriate time is marriage.

Is it OK for me to have the urge to masturbate?

An urge for anything can be normal. How we respond is an issue of applying our values and beliefs to that urge. When someone has the urge to masturbate, the real question might be how to respond. See question

#1. Sexual urges are not, in and of themselves, sinful, unless you feed them to the point of looking at pornography, stimulating yourself sexually (masturbating), engaging in heavy petting, or lustfully drinking someone in with your eyes. So the urge to masturbate is common. Ask yourself how following Jesus impacts what you do with that urge.

How do I say no to sex?

Motivation is usually the key to maintaining purity and saying no to sex or to any other sin. First of all, not having sex can be very challenging for some, especially if you stay in situations where arousal has been stirred. The urges are strong. To answer your question in brief (see chapter nine for more details), talking with a mentor openly about your desire for sex is a key component to figuring out how to say no. Also, how is your understanding of the scriptures in this area? Do you know how to find them? Do you read them and meditate on them? Being deeply rooted in God's Word is vital. You may have received some pat or trite answers to this in the past and it is important to have convictions that are solidly based on Scripture. Finally, what is your dream for a relationship? Some people find it helpful to keep a journal in which they write to their future spouse. They tell their spouse about the ways they are preparing themselves to be their partner and the hopes and dreams they have for their marriage to them.

How do I resist the temptation to fantasize?

Pictures are everywhere. As this is being typed, our Yahoo Mail site has a pop-up picture of a woman in a bra. Argh! In our chapter nine on *Purity and Holiness* we talk about making the object of your fantasy into a person. Go take a closer look at what that means. Also, have a specific action plan on what you are going to do when you are pulled toward fantasy. If you struggle with habitual unwanted fantasies, repression (wishing they would stop) usually doesn't help. Instead, confront the fantasy head on and ask Jesus to come help you figure it out. What does it mean? What would Jesus do if He were there? A great book to read is Stephanie Carnes', *The Fantasy Fallacy*.

So ask yourself, do you have a plan? A plan could consist of who you are going to call, having specific Scriptures to help you out, and knowing what kind of physical activity you're going to do instead (send a text to someone to encourage them, go on a prayer walk, cook a new recipe, go pound some nails). Have a plan. Share it with someone. When you don't follow it, when you blow it, tell someone you trust and have them hold you accountable. Adjust your plan whenever needed in order to find the best ways to keep your heart and mind where God wants them.

Am I sinful if I dream about having sex, even though I am not actually having sex?

Though popular literature might tell you otherwise, we usually cannot control what we dream about. Now, obviously, if we indulge in pornography, watch shows with sexual innuendos or sexual relationships, read romance novels, and watch chick flicks, it can absolutely affect our dreams. The dream is not the sin, but could be fueled by sexual stimulation while you are awake. If you have an intense sexual dream and can't pinpoint where it came from, it can be very disturbing. Talk to someone. Share it. Do not let embarrassment stop you. The only power Satan has is if we keep in the dark what we are going through, even when what we are experiencing is not necessarily sin.

How do I overcome my physical desires as a single parent?

Unless you adopted a child, being a parent means you had sex either before marriage or during marriage. You may have become single after a divorce or the death of a spouse. Some single parents never married. In any case, you may miss having sex. You may miss the body-to-body intimacy. You may still long for the warmth of another body to wake up to, to cuddle with, and to kiss, and the pleasure of sex and orgasm. You still have those desires. When desire comes, you may want so badly to *overcome* the desire that you push it away. We recommend a different approach.

When you feel the desire rise up in you, notice it. It is natural. Squishing it down may not be the best course of action. Notice it and accept it. You may need to mourn the loss. Sex is enjoyable and you are missing it. That is understandable. From that point, your values can direct what to do from there. If the desire is connected with wanting to arouse yourself with self-stimulation and this is not compatible with what you believe, have a plan (see question #4). Remember, when we make the decision to submit our body to God, the very process of submitting is putting ourselves into the presence of God in order to allow Him to work on our very heart and character. For further on this, we recommend *Celebration of Discipline* by Richard Foster.

It may help to take some time to journal what you are feeling. Then speak openly with a friend. Most likely, someone else has the same feelings and they can relate. So notice it, accept it, share it, and then pray. God calls us to bring all our hopes and desires to Him (Psalms 130:7, Philippians 4:6). You may also be in need of godly physical affection. Talk about this with friends and those you are close to. By pushing through any awkwardness, you may be surprised to find your friends feel the same need. Finally, check and see if what you are truly looking for is close companionship. Making sure that you have close, deep relationships is vital to sexual purity.

Is it wrong for me to want to have a companion?

God made us to be in intimately connected. Psalm 139 says that He knows our thoughts, discerns when we lay down, and created our innermost parts. Through the prophet Isaiah, God calls us beloved, tells us that we are engraved on the palm of His hand, reminds us that He carries us close to His heart, and says, possessively, "You are mine!" (Isaiah 40:11, 43:1, 49:16). God also created us to be intimately connected to others. "It is not good for man to be alone. I will make a helper suitable for him" (Genesis 2:18). Wanting to be with someone intimately—mind, emotions, soul and body—absolutely falls within God's plan. What is hard is when we do not know if it is in His plan for us and whether it will *happen*. You have probably heard many different answers about trusting God with the timing, and loving being single. To answer your specific question, we would add that you are created to want someone. That desire is normal and beautiful. Then take that desire before the God who knows our hearts and our desires and who does have great plans for us.

Is it acceptable to have physical intimacy with someone and not be in a committed relationship?

What a good question. We would encourage you to look at chapter nine, *Purity and Holiness.* If you are intimate with someone that you are not committed to in any form (not dating or engaged), you may want to ask yourself why you are being physically intimate and whether that is best for that relationship. Are you considering what is best for them (Philippians 2:3-4)? Are you doing things physically that are causing arousal and giving Satan a foothold (Ephesians 4:7)? Are you creating expectations in yourself or the other with the physical intimacy? Probably. Also, it also depends on what type of physical touch we are talking about. 1 Corinthians 12 teaches us that there are certain parts of our body that are unpresentable. Any touching of the genitals would be considered sexual by any standard. However, even touch to non-sexual parts of the body can be very arousing. And touch to the genitals, even when there is a barrier of clothing, is arousing and can lead to orgasm. Consider these things as you are making decisions.

If someone was sexually active before becoming a Christian, but no longer experiences any urge for sex since, is that normal? Is it normal that now that I'm older, I don't struggle with the temptation to masturbate? And will this affect my future if I get married?

There are some who might call that a blessing to not be tempted to masturbate. However, the reality is, sexual interest (or sexual urges, sexual libido, sexual desire) can ebb and flow. Some people feel urges for sex daily. Others not at all. And then there is everything in between. There are those who would say that not feeling any sexual urge must mean something is not normal. "Normal" is a challenging word and it's possible there are perfectly good reasons that someone is not interested in sex. If sex was violating, unfulfilling, or not enjoyable, that can definitely make someone uninterested in having sex. If someone has a background where they were sexually abused, this can lower their interest in sex even when they had more of an interest in earlier relationships. However, when people lead busy, productive lives and they are doing things that are fulfilling and meaningful, the level of missing sex can be remarkably low. Most people find that when they once again enter a loving marriage relationship based on God where they are both genuinely giving, they have a mutually enjoyable sexual relationship.

How do I deal with the fact that I feel validated when others find me physically attractive?

For many men and women, knowing someone is physically attracted to them makes them feel more confident. It's pretty normal to enjoy looking good. However, this can also be problematic. If we get our confidence from how we look, this can then mean that we do not feel secure unless we look good. This leaves our security dependent on the approval of others, and that can be a real snare. "The fear of man can be a snare" (Proverbs 29:25). Women who are naturally beautiful can also become quite insecure about their looks especially as they age. They often share that they worry about the loss of something that gave them confidence for so long. Recognizing beauty and enjoying it is one thing but depending on it for security can be problematic. Also, it is true that when couples base their relationship on physical attraction, rather than on God and on being spiritually attracted to one another, the relationship can have any number of challenges. It helps to remember that God calls women to be primarily focused on having a *character* that is beautiful. "Your beauty should not come from outward adornment, such as elaborate hairstyles and the wearing of gold jewelry or fine clothes. Rather, it should be that of your inner self, the unfading beauty of a gentle and quiet spirit, which is of great worth in God's sight" (1 Peter 3:3-4). We would say be amazed by the body that God created because it is fearfully and wonderfully made (Psalm 139:14). And then use that body to serve others and serve God. The genuine validation that works long term is validation from God who takes delight in us. You can both embrace your attractive physical appearance and not be focused on it or use it to make yourself feel more validated as a person. A great book to address this is *Secure in Heart*, by Robin Weidner.

I started doing pornography as a fourteen-year-old, and then had early experiences of sex. How do I correct the thoughts that still go through my head?

Ah yes, can the brain be corrected and rewired? First of all, read chapter ten on *Masturbation and Pornography*. Correcting the thoughts that go through the head can be an uphill climb where pornography is concerned, and it takes someone making radical, consistent decisions to get there. Because the use of pornography and masturbation involves sight, physical sensations, and emotions, the emotional reward system of the body can lay down tracks pretty deeply. Again, it is critical to have an action plan. Make one. In that plan, have specific things you are going to do when you are pulled to think those thoughts. Get someone you trust to hold you accountable, make sure you do lots of other rewarding things in your life, and get radical about replacing the thoughts and actions with other thoughts and actions. One of the primary ways we recommend correcting thoughts is whenever you are drawn to dwelling on sexual pictures in your head, remember that that woman or man you're think-ing about is a person (see the chapter *Masturbation and Pornography*). God is the Creator of your body and your heart. Ask Him to help you with literally rerouting your heart and brain. He can. He made you. Just make sure you do your part.

How do I deal with the temptations to masturbate that I cannot escape?

This is such an honest question and we answered most of it above. However, there is one more consideration. "No temptation has overtaken you except what is common to mankind. And God is faithful; he will not let you be tempted beyond what you can bear. But when you are tempted, he will also provide a way out so that you can endure it" (1 Corinthians 10:13). Let's be honest. Most of the time when people say they don't have a way out, it is because they have not worked hard yet at setting up a good escape plan. And you need to get someone to help you. You can escape. Scripture says you can. Remember, most of the time, sexual temptation is like a wave that you need to ride. You are able to ride that wave, without taking any action to respond by doing something sexually. Ride the wave and eventually the pull subsides. But you will need lots of help along the ride. You can escape. You just need to make sure you have a really effective escape plan already set up and a trustworthy friend to walk that journey with you.

Is it wrong that I stop myself from falling into temptation by saying to myself that if I do it, something bad will happen to me?

Motivation is such a huge part of how we deal with sin. Fear is definitely a motivator. So is happiness, grace, and joy. So are bad consequences and punishment. None of these in and of themselves are bad motivators. However, most of these by themselves won't last very long and after a while, people learn to live with a surprising amount of bad consequences. The main problem with psyching yourself out with the possibility that something bad could happen is that you are going to figure out eventually that what happens might not seem all that bad to you. It really depends on your definition of bad. If you masturbate or have sex, you could feel shame. You could damage your relationship with God or with someone else. You could wire your brain to get used to your hand. You could feel guilty and quit praying to God. And yes, you could get someone pregnant or get a sexual disease. So yes, something bad could happen. However, you probably won't get hit by a car and a lightning bolt probably won't come down from heaven. And if you masturbate, though it could have any number of negative consequences, you can still go to heaven. It is so important to remember that the goal of someone in love with God is to honor Him with their body, to flee sexual immorality, to live a life of love, and to show people the wonder of who God is. Remember, "Grace ... teaches us to say no to ungodliness and worldly passions, and to live self-controlled, upright and godly lives in this present age" (Titus 2:12). That kind of motivation will probably last a bit longer and be much more fulfilling.

Is it wrong or impure for a dating couple to hold hands when they talk and pray together?

Those who are dating make a lot of different decisions on how much affection and touch to engage in. There are some kinds of touches that cause arousal that can then make staying pure in thought and deed a bit difficult. Holding hands wouldn't typically fall under that category, though you can definitely talk about it, both between you and your boyfriend or girlfriend and with those involved in your life (a teen or singles ministry leader, etc.). However, healthy, affectionate touch is a good way to draw closer and to figure out if this is someone you would want to have a more committed relationship with. I (Jennifer) have a wonderful, distinct memory of the first time Tim and I held hands walking through Balboa Park here in San Diego. Being able to hold hands with him brought me so much joy. I can still feel the huge grin on my face. I loved feeling his fingers wrapped around mine and feeling his thumb as it lightly passed over my knuckles (our kids are going "ewwww" right now). You don't hold hands that way with just anyone, and when you get to do that with someone you love, it can be the most wonderful thing.

Once pornography is in your mind, how do you get rid of it? How do I overcome seeing sexual images or even seeing images of people's private parts?

Yes, once those pictures are in there, it is hard to get rid of them. Like a pop-up ad on Yahoo, pictures you don't wish to look at will just pop up in your mind. This is especially true for those who have looked at a lot of them on the Internet. In fact, sometimes it can feel like the images flood you. When we experience something, and when that memory has a distinct emotion and picture attached to it (such as heart pounding excitement), even when we no longer want to have that memory in our brain, it can be very persistent.

Most of the time—just like the decision not to continue looking at the pop-up on Yahoo and not to take that second look at someone walking by—the first step is to make that covenant with your eyes and with your mind not to dwell on the thought. Guy Hammond has a wonderful book called *Tempt Away*. Get it. He approaches what to do with those lightning pictures and thoughts in an honest, humorous, real way. Basically, though the thoughts are going to come, with consistent prayer and openness, they come less over time. This is similar to the challenge for those who used to use bad language a lot before they became a Christian. It can be hard to overcome the automatic response of letting that word come out. However, God is a God of miracles. Ask Him to help you with your brain. Accept that the pictures will still pop up, but when they do, plan ahead of time what you're going to do.

Consider this example from Michelle Smith, author of *Prodigal Pursued*. She shares how an ancient author advised that one should "turn the mind [away from the impure thought] to some spiritual, or, at least, *indifferent object*. It is useful to combat other bad thoughts face to face, but not thoughts of impurity."

Smith then shares her own example, saying, "I started turning my thoughts to something else entirely. This is a skill, like serving a volleyball or balancing a tray, and it takes practice. In the beginning, all I could do was literally move my eyes to an inanimate object and start mentally describing it. 'The vase is slender, blue, glass. The flower is yellow.' As I continued to practice, I could eventually call forth scripture or envision the cross. I learned not to linger, not to try to get a little enjoyment out of the image or thought before turning my attention, but to do so immediately."

So find a simple practice to engage in when the thought flashes through and put it into practice again and again. Pray. Read Scripture. Do the practice every time. Be open with someone about it, and then watch God work.

How do I talk to my parents about sex?

Well, ask them to prayerfully consider reading *Redeemed Sexuality*. Seriously. Most parents feel incredibly uncomfortable talking about sex. Their own parents didn't do it well. Your parents probably have their own hang-ups in regards to sex. They have their own shame.

But that's not just true of parents. Doctors, who are trained to include sexual questions when they do a checkup, rarely ask them. Even therapists, who are more specifically trained to ask about sexuality, often do not. Parents, though that is their job, are often really uncomfortable too. So bring it up. Have them read the chapters in *Redeemed Sexuality* that you find most helpful, then talk together about it. Taking those steps can sometimes get the process started. And if your parent just does not have it in them to have more of a conversation, find someone you trust who will. Plus, you can email us at theartofintimatemarriage@yahoo.com. We'd love to talk with you.

What is the best conversation opener to talk about same gender sex when talking to parents?

It is truly unfortunate when a young man or woman struggles with same-sex attraction, or with wondering about their sexual attractions ("Am I bisexual, asexual, gay, lesbian?") and doesn't have a place to talk about it. If you want to talk openly with your parent, have them read the chapter on *Sexual Identity Development* and then say you would like to discuss it together. You can do this as well with anyone you want to have this kind of conversation with. Even if you are not same-sex attracted, you may have a lot of questions and want to talk with your parents. Sometimes it helps to start with discussing a character that might be in a show you're watching and going from there. If you are an adult helping other parents, have them read the chapter mentioned in this paragraph, or even better, read it along with them and have a great time talking.

How do I avoid lustful thoughts toward women at church (from a single brother)? How tempting is it for brothers if we do not pay attention to the way we dress (from a sister)?

For the brothers, we suggest you first check how your thoughts are going toward all women. Douglas Rosenau suggests making any woman you are tempted to think lustful thoughts about into a person. See more on this in chapter nine. However, at church, relationships can be closer and more intimate. There may be times where touch can be more personal. Also, not every sister dresses as they should and that may be something to address in your congregation. Sisters, are you helping each other with how you dress, helping one another to be considerate? Men, consider Paul's advice to Timothy. "Treat... younger women as sisters, with absolute purity" (1 Timothy 5:2). That woman is a sister in Christ and worthy of honor. Treat her with honor. Do not allow your thoughts to linger on her body. Remember her as a person. Also, remember she is going to perhaps be someone's wife one day. And there is possibly another woman out there who is going to be your wife one day. How would you want the brothers to think about her? If you have a daughter one day, how would you want the men at church to think about here? Our lives are bigger than the individual moments, and it can help to remember the bigger picture.

How do I get away from doing pornography when each time I keep saying it is the last time?

When someone has repeatedly said, "This is the last time" and then they do it again, it is possible that they have developed an addiction to something. I (Jennifer) am not particularly fond of the word addiction, though I am actually an addictions counselor. However, the word can be useful in putting a name to what they are experiencing and how to overcome something. The markers for having an addiction are the following:

1. Doing or taking something in larger amounts or for a longer time than intended;
2. Wanting to cut down or quit and not being able to;
3. Spending a lot of time setting up for or obtaining it;
4. Craving it or having a strong desire for it;
5. Continuing to do it even when there are negative consequences at work, at school, in your relationships, or with your health;
6. Needing to take or do an increased amount in order to experience the high, the excitement, the euphoria (with sexual addiction this means doing it more often and looking at increasingly more graphic material); and,
7. Feeling symptoms of withdrawal or feelings of irritation and agitation when you have not done it for a while.

To qualify for a diagnosis of addiction, you need two to three of these. For most, recognizing how serious a problem they have is the first step in overcoming it. Consider getting more support, such as joining a support program, getting a mentor or sponsor, and seeing someone professionally to figure out if there are underlying reasons why you are turning to pornography. Most of the time, people have to do a mixture of radically working on their relationship with God, radically opening up their life, working closely with a mentor, and getting good group support for the process of recovery.

Is marriage meant for procreation?

Obviously marriage can lead to having babies and babies can come without marriage. God does say in Genesis, "Be fruitful and multiply" (Genesis 1:28). And the only place the Scriptures teach to have sex and children is within marriage. However, there are many other wonderful things that marriage is also for. Marriage shows us, in a very concrete way, what the relationship is between Christ and His bride. The entire Bible is a book on that marriage. Marriage is also about showing love, serving one another, submitting to one another, and enjoying an intimate connection. Dave and Judy Weger did our premarital counseling, and Dave had always said that when you consider someone to marry, choose someone who will be your partner in the Gospel and who will help you get to heaven. Marriage can be an amazing spiritual partnership.

The variation of this question we most commonly hear is similar: "Is sex meant for procreation?" Sex can cause procreation. It can lead to children being born. However, sex is also meant to be pleasurable. The greatest number of nerves in the body are found in the genitals. God intended sex to feel good. God also intended for marriage and sex to make two people one flesh (Genesis 2:24). And sometimes that leads to children. In early church history, there was a teaching for a long time that the only purpose of sex was for procreation. In Genesis 1:28, God does in fact tell Adam and Eve to be fruitful and multiply, filling the earth. However, the Scriptures, especially Song of Songs, make it very clear that God designed sex also for enjoyment in order for a husband and wife to have a beautiful, fun, erotic connection between them.

What is the line between sexual arousal and lust?

The word in Matthew 5:28, "Do not look at a woman with lust" is *epithumeo*, which means focused on, or to desire, covet, lust, set the heart upon something with a passionate desire. This kind of focus or desire can actually be on anything, such as money, food, or drink. However, in this passage and others, the desire is sexual and it is toward a woman. In the Greek, this word is stronger than we hear it in English. This is not just a passing glance. This is not just a wish. This is a continued gaze that should be elsewhere.

Sexual arousal can also be connected to lust, but there can be different scenarios. There are times when someone looks at someone or something and they feel an instantaneous arousal (this would be like the knee-jerk reaction talked about in the Arousal and Orgasm section of chapter eight, *Sexual Anatomy 101*). They might look away quickly and not lust, but they have still experienced arousal. They can then choose not to linger or take a second look, and allow their body to gradually return to its unaroused state. However, there are other times where someone lusts, by taking that continued time to look, and then arousal happens. So there isn't necessarily a clear line between arousal and lust. However, if someone does not respond to their arousal in a God-pleasing manner, their arousal can then become entwined with lust and lead to sin. Enticement, or arousal, is not necessarily sin. Aim to draw a line that keeps you from being drawn away (James 1:14). To linger. To pursue. To lust. Once you draw that line, don't even get close to it. If the enticement or arousal comes up, have a good plan in mind to deal with it. And don't put yourself in situations when you will have a higher chance of crossing that line (i.e., the alcoholic going into a bar is like the young person going on their computer later at night to surf the web; not always a wise choice since web surfing at night can often lead to using pornography).

If arousal is considered natural, how do you make sure that it is guided by God and not be tempted by Satan? If sexual arousal is normal, but doesn't feel right, how do you overcome that thought? Are there ways to control it?

The ways that our body responds to sexual cues are God-given responses. God created sexual arousal to help prepare the body for sexual intimacy in marriage. There are a number of ways to bring God into this intimate part of your life. Refrain from doing things that intentionally cause arousal. However, if arousal happens spontaneously, notice what a good job God did in making the body. Next, take that arousal to God and consider what He wants you to do with it. If you are single, that would mean choosing not to feed it or pursue the temptation to do something sexual.

Satan is the master of deceit, the father of lies. He takes everything that is good and twists it. The tree of life was good, but God said don't eat of it or you will die. Satan came and took those godly instructions and twisted God's words and said, "Surely you will not die ... God knows that when you eat it, your eyes will be opened" (Genesis 3:4-5). Well, Adam and Eve's eyes were definitely opened. The reality is, in the same way, Satan takes sexuality, which is beautiful and good, and puts it into pornography, puts it into adulterous relationships, draws people to violate others with it, and lures people to have it before they should. And Satan also seeks ways to use the God-given physiological response of sexual arousal against us. He either tempts us to indulge it before we should, tells us that we might as well indulge since we've already sinned, or tells us we should feel guilty even when we process it in a pure way. Remember, just like your glands salivating doesn't mean you should necessarily have that whole bag of chips, that God-given physiological arousal response does not mean you should just go have sex. And just because your glands salivated thinking of those chips doesn't mean you need to feel guilty for the way God made your body.

Remember, the sexual response itself is not necessarily sin, but pursuing that response with sexual action—with people, at times, or in ways that God does not intend—is.

Since masturbation and pornography are quite rampant for brothers, how do you really overcome it?

How we overcome masturbation and pornography is covered above, so we want to address one part of this question here. There is a common belief that masturbation and pornography is more of a brother thing, more of a guy thing. However, research shows us that, although the percentage is definitely higher for men, 30 percent of women also struggle with viewing pornography and masturbating. Women also need the support, accountability, and direction that men do.

Since sexuality is beautiful and a God-made phenomenon to be enjoyed in marriage, how, as a single individual, can I be pure while still having a healthy, spiritual view of sexuality and not feel like I'm trying to suppress or kill my sexuality?

One of the first things you'll really want to do is examine your view of purity. If you see it as a drag, it will be very difficult to enjoy and appreciate purity. Hopefully, reading this book will help you get there. Many singles report wondering whether righteousness requires them to suppress or kill their sexuality. Good luck. That would mean you would have to literally die. You are a sexual person. It is vital that each of us believes and embraces that. Like money, sexuality is a gift from God and we are called to steward it well. We would recommend seeing it that way. Rather than trying to suppress or kill it, remember God has made you a steward of your body and your sexuality. If one day God chooses to give you someone with whom to live out that stewardship together, it will be a beautiful opportunity to use that gift to give joy to your spouse.

How do I stop the desire to watch loving, sexual dramas?

We so appreciate this question. This comes from someone who realizes that it isn't just pornography that is sinful. Sexual dramas, movies, TV shows, books, or romance novels with sex scenes are commonly called soft porn, and rightly so. One of the important things is to call something what it is. If you are drawn to reading or watching things that have sex in them, this is not much different from someone going onto the internet and watching pornography. Know that even if you desire to watch these kinds of shows, that doesn't mean you have to pursue the desire. First of all, check your biblical convictions about sex and your overall heart and desire to say no to sin because of your gratitude for the sake of the cross. Ask yourself how your hunger and thirst for righteousness is going (Matthew 6:5). Secondly, examine what are you getting out of these shows. People pursue sexual stimulation for many different reasons. It gives them a sexual rush. It takes them away from their unhappiness. It lowers their stress for a short time. They feel it's fun. If you don't examine what you're getting out of it, it may be hard to stop. Look at the underlying factors pulling you toward this and ask yourself honestly whether sexuality was intended for this purpose.

Finally, as mentioned above, make a plan. Be open with what you are struggling with and get someone to hold you accountable. God does have the power to change what draws our heart and mind, but we have to do our part. Get radical about this and see what God can do.

I know the Bible teaches we are not supposed to have sex until we are married. I did, though, and I still feel guilty in God. What should I do?

Guilt is a natural response to seeing our sin before God. God calls us to feel guilt and Paul even says that godly sorrow is necessary for change (1 Corinthians 7:10). We are often told that we should not feel shame. However, the Bible clearly teaches that not feeling shame and not blushing when we look at our sin is quite a problem (Jeremiah 6:15).

However, we are also called to rejoice in God's grace and to relish His forgiveness every morning. In fact, when we repent, the Scriptures tell us that our sins have been "wiped out" and that we can now experience "times of refreshing" (Acts 3:19). It can be particularly hard to feel that our sexual sin has been wiped out. The level of guilt can be higher often because sex overall seems so much more shameful.

However, that is not the view that God has. In fact, when Jesus was with women who had committed sexual sin, we see Him being compassionate, loving, and warm (John 4 and John 8). And when they publicly expressed their sorrow for their sin, we see Him holding them up as incredible examples (Luke 7:44-50). You may need to reevaluate your understanding of God's heart toward your sexual sin. God does hate sin and He did tell the woman caught in adultery to leave her life of sin. He also held up a prostitute as an example of someone who loved much, a woman so grateful for Jesus that she wept at His feet and washed His feet with her hair. He told her to "Go in peace." His forgiveness should leave us with peace. Jesus reserves his sharpest rebukes for the religiously prideful. He shows some of His greatest compassion toward those who have sexually sinned. Perhaps we should imitate Him. Take some significant time to meditate upon these scriptures and ask God to help you understand His heart toward you.

What are the Christian/biblical guidelines about BDSM?

Well, you just asked that, didn't you? And we will tell you, this is not just a question that married individuals ask. Christian singles sometimes know more about *Fifty Shades of Grey* than their parents. Because we do not want to put any more pictures in your mind than might already be warring within you, let us respond with this. When we work with married couples, they often have questions about what they should include in their sex life. We give them a What's Allowed list and encourage them to consider together the activity one of them wants to include and to come to a decision together. We include it here so that you understand, even before marriage, how a couple can talk through some of these questions (a version of this is included for engaged couples in the chapter *Save Yourself*). We hope this is helpful.

What's Allowed: Eight Questions to Guide Your Sexual Choices in Marriage

1. Is it prohibited by Scripture (i.e., lust, sexual immorality: Matthew 5:28, Galatians 5:19-21)?
2. Is it beneficial and constructive (1 Corinthians 10:23-24)? Does it build up? Does it benefit your relationship, and are you seeking your spouse's good?
3. Does it involve anyone else (including fantasizing—Hebrews 13:4, Matthew 5:28)?
4. What is the fruit (Matthew 7:16-20)? When you put it into practice, does it create intimate connection between you? Does it lead to anything detrimental?
5. Is it too contaminated by pollution of the world (James 1:27) or has Satan contaminated it but now it needs to be reclaimed (2 Peter 1:3-4)?
6. Is it pleasing to your spouse (1 Corinthians 7:33-34)?

7. Does it violate your or your spouse's conscience (Romans 14:5, 1 Corinthians 8:7-13)?

8. If you choose not to engage in this, is it truly about restraining or controlling sensual/sexual corruption in a God-given manner, or is it based on human teachings and self-imposed, false restrictions of the body (Colossians 2:21-23)?

Is it normal to get "wet" from kissing/making out?

Kissing and making out can definitely get the juices flowing. Getting wet is usually the term used to describe the result of sexual arousal in women when the natural lubrication of the vagina is secreted. It would actually be the equivalent of the penis becoming erect. Some people kiss and do not become erect or wet. Most people become wet or erect when they make out. It is normal. Is it best? That is probably the real question. If someone is engaging in something that is causing that level of a sexual response, it may be time to look at how their healthy boundaries are. Petting, making out, and heavy kissing can awaken and arouse love before its time (Song of Songs 2:7). Check out chapters nine and twelve on *Purity and Holiness* and *Save Yourself* as you determine what you want to continue doing in your physical intimacy before you get married.

Since sexual arousal is a natural reaction, what can someone who is single do to 'pacify' themselves?

We have covered how to respond to sexual arousal; however, we want to answer one other part here. The need to pacify. Sometimes what someone is asking is whether there is some kind of sexual outlet that is appropriate. Most of the time, though, people want to know how to calm that need. The first thing we recommend is accept the bodily response. Sometimes just accepting the body for what it is and choosing not to act on it is the primary step. Also, this may be an opportunity to consider what are some other real needs you have that are that are not sexual but that sometimes express themselves through sexual arousal. You may have a need for rest, relaxation, relief from stress, something entertaining, or something fun. So check that. What you need to pacify may not be the need for sex but rather the need for recreation, the need for fun, or the need for affectionate connection. Pacify that! Then accept your body as it is while giving your sexual response over to God.

How can dating couples be intimate physically but still stay within healthy boundaries? It feels taboo to even talk about it and should dating couples kiss?

We have covered this pretty thoroughly in our chapters in *Purity and Holiness* and *Save Yourself.* In our ministries, we can make it very difficult for people to feel that they can come and talk about their temptations. We need to make sure we are not making things taboo and, instead, provide our singles with an atmosphere in which they can ask their questions without fear of condemnation.

So, how would that look for those being asked? Listen. Listen some more. Ask questions. Not questions that are like an interrogation ("How dare you do that?" or "How could you have gotten yourself into that situation?"). Ask questions that seek to understand what is happening and how they are feeling about it. "The purposes of a person's heart are deep waters, but a man or woman of understanding draws them out" (Proverbs 20:5). Explore their doubts with them and point them to the Scriptures. Above, we share a question one single/teen had, "Should dating couples kiss?" As tempting as it might be to tell them what they should do, take the time to explore what they are hearing, thinking, and considering.

How would that look for those asking? Make sure you pray before you ask for advice. Pray that God will use those you are asking and that God will give them wisdom to guide you. Pray for humility and a surrendered heart. And make sure if you have any feelings about how your questions are answered (the tone, any disagreement, further doubts or wonderings), make sure you talk some more.

What are the ramifications of a person that's had too much explanation and discussions about sexuality with your parent(s) and seeing your parents commit adultery/having sex with someone other than their wife/husband?

There are times when parents over-explain or talk about sexuality in a way that feels intrusive to their children. Some parents make sexual jokes or share too much information about their own sexual activities or the issues they have in their marital sexual relationship. Other parents engage in extramarital relationships either before or during marriage. These kinds of experiences can cause a number of difficulties for someone. Both Jennifer and I experienced some of these challenges. It is actually common that people do. If your parent did any of these things, you may have a negative view of sex or you may have a wrong understanding of what sex is supposed to be like. You may have some resentment and anger about choices your parents made. When you get married, you may need to work through a number of challenges affected by those choices. These experiences can taint your experience and view of sex, and cause problems with sexual demands, sexual functioning, and sexual inhibition. They can also lead to sexual promiscuity or to the opposite, an aversion for sex. We would first of all recommend that you speak openly with someone you trust about these experiences and possibly speak with someone professionally. When you do get married, read the chapter on *Families and Sexuality* together and share your thoughts. Pray and seek guidance. And remember, God can make all things new.

What do you do when you are physically/sexually attracted to a brother you are building a relationship with or have an interest in? What's a good way to defer/address this feeling?

Physical attraction is usually about finding someone physically attractive (handsome or beautiful) and/or feeling the desire to look at and admire their body (i.e., their shape, form, breasts, buttocks, muscles, etc.). Sexual attraction is often more about wanting to touch, kiss, and sexually be with someone. It may mean feeling your body becoming aroused when you think about or see that person. These feelings are normal and natural. However, lingering on them can be problematic and can cause someone to be more excited about the physical part of a relationship than the emotional and spiritual part of a relationship. It is normal to feel these things, but letting these feelings guide your decisions about your relationship can cause any number of unwise choices (such as sexual impurity and sexual immorality), or can cause couples to move their relationship forward much more quickly than may be best for them.

We also recommend that you listen to the Psalmist: "Charm is deceptive, and beauty is fleeting; but a woman who fears the LORD is to be praised" (Psalm 31:30). Let's reword this for the brothers. "Charm is deceptive, and a handsome face and body is fleeting; but a man who fears the LORD is to be praised." Good looks may not always endure. Build your relationships and your future family wisely by focusing your mind on that brother's or sister's fear and love for God.

"I believe in liberal sex: sex is natural so do it with love and responsibility. Why is this wrong?"

This one could use a whole chapter. However, we wanted to include a short answer here because this is such a huge question for those who are teens and singles today. There is a common belief that if you love someone and if you are not harming anyone, then sexual relationships are good and right. There are some within different churches that teach this. Let us answer two different things here; one about love, and one about harm.

Love is not just about emotion. "This is how we know that we love the children of God: by loving God and carrying out his commands" (1 John 5:2). If you love the person you are with, you will be more concerned with what is best for their relationship with God more than you will about having sex with them. We need to define love as God defines it. According to this scripture, if you truly love someone, you will carry out the commands of God, not just follow your own wishes, desires, and feelings. Someone's eternity and their relationship with God will be of paramount importance to you. Remember, people can love someone and have sex with them even when the relationship is completely inappropriate (i.e., someone else's spouse). An emotional feeling of love is not the only standard that someone who trusts God would use to make a decision about whether to engage sexually.

We also need to see what we define as harm. Research has shown that sex in uncommitted relationships has negative consequences.[1] It is also important to note how we define harm. Read chapter eleven, *The Body is Not Made for Sexual Immorality* which details some of the physical, emotional, and spiritual harms that come with sexual immorality.

God made us. He adores us. He doesn't make up rules to harm us. "For I know the plans I have for you. Plans to prosper you and not to harm you. Plans to give you a hope and a future" (Jeremiah 29:11). When God gives us boundaries for our sexual choices, He does so because He knows what is best for us and what can harm us. Trust Him.

"If being sexually active before becoming a disciple, what can one do as a single woman when our biological instincts occur/arousal and help in remaining pure?"

You may have woken love up before God intended (Song of Songs 8:4). Your body knows what it is like to have an orgasm and sometimes you feel the pull and the arousal rise up in you. What do you do? We mostly address this in earlier chapters. However, we want to answer one part of this question here. There are physiological results to things we engaged in before becoming a Christian. Our bodies create habits and can become accustomed to any number of things. Some of the greatest pulls are smoking and drug use, alcohol, overeating, masturbation, and sex. Read James 1:14. Some of our desires are not from God and can lead to sin and death if we indulge them. However, James makes an important

---

[1]   Willis, S. R. (2011). The relationship between pre-marital sexual activity and subsequent marital dissolution. Dissertation Abstracts International Section A, 72, 1461

point in this scripture and the word he uses is *enticed*. The enticement to engage in sex is often going to be stronger because we have engaged in it sooner than we should have. However, it is vital that we give room for the reality of enticement. It is not at that point that someone has sinned. But it is at that point that someone needs to be open with what they are feeling. Be open with your enticements. They are understandable and real. Then allow your openness to lead you to a washing in the blood and a fellowship with one another. "If we walk in the light, as he is in the light, we have fellowship with one another, and the blood of Jesus, his Son, purifies us from all sin" (1 John 1:7).

How do you maintain purity after so many years of giving your all to God? And still trust that you can be married.

You may have heard many different answers to this question. In fact, some of those answers can sound like being chaste, remaining pure, is easy. And that kind of dismissive response can be frustrating and discouraging. We want to make a few points here. Lauren Winner in *Real Sex* and Matthew Anderson in *Earthen Vessels* both make a strong point about how our view of human sexuality must be deeply embedded in God's vision for humankind's bodies. So first of all, to maintain purity over years, you may want to place your practice of purity within the broader context of your practice of bodily living (see chapter eleven). You may or may not ever marry. However, finding good robust ways to live bodily is so important regardless. Dance. Hike. Play in the ocean. Hug your friends. Feel the water of a river on your skin. Do yoga. Enjoy a softball or soccer game. Ride a bike. Hug a friend again. Turn on the music and dance. Climb a mountain and hike to a waterfall. An incredibly important part of maintaining a celibate life is living passionately in the body you have.

There is a common teaching that sex is essential to a man's flourishing; however, most would say that this is true only for a married man. Hmm .... where does that leave the single men among us? So we ask you to consider that another important way to maintain sexual purity over many years is by taking on a different view of sex overall. Our flourishing is not dependent on having sex, whether we are married or single. Married brothers, if you are counseling single brothers in their purity, examine your own beliefs in this.

Finally, consider the importance of practicing some of the spiritual disciplines such as prayer, fasting, study of the Word, meditation, worship, service, and confession. We engage in these disciplines in order to place ourselves in the presence of God so that He can transform us. "He who sows to the Spirit will from the Spirit reap eternal life" (Galatians 6:8). As Foster says in *Celebration of Discipline*, when we want to grow something, we plant it, cultivate it, and water it, but then the "natural forces of the earth take over and up comes the grain" (p. 7). This is exactly how sexual discipline works. We engage in it in order to place ourselves before God so that He can take us to a place where transformation can occur. Whether someone is single or married, whether they marry one day or never marry, the practice of sexual discipline is important.

So to maintain purity through the years, take the broader view of what you are engaging in; living bodily in Christ, flourishing without sex, and growing through the spiritual disciplines including sexual discipline. To answer the last part of this question, you may marry one day or you may not marry. God makes no promises. He does, however, promise life to the full, so surrender your life to God and find out what that means for you.

My boyfriend struggles with addiction to pornography. How as a girlfriend can I help in his fight? Is there anything that I can or cannot do?

We applaud you for asking this question. At times, during dating and engagement, a boyfriend or girlfriend finds out that the person they love struggles with pornography. It can be pretty scary and sometimes people wonder if they should stay together. There are ways to be supportive. You can do this by encouraging a boyfriend or girlfriend to seek help. Be honest with them about your convictions. Also, do your own work in understanding this problem. Talk with those to whom you are close and to others who are experienced in dealing with these kinds of challenges. If you find that there is a lot of deceit and hiding happening, this may be a time to emphasize the importance of seeking significant help and where you may need to take a stand on the future of your relationship.

There can be some problematic responses to be aware of. There are some who decide that in order to help their partner stay away from pornography, they will engage with them sexually. Using sex to keep someone from doing pornography doesn't work. Not only does this mean that you will be engaging in sex outside of God's plan, this kind of sex leads to resentment, anger, and frustration and it does not lead to learning healthy sexuality. In the language of the recovery movement, your boyfriend or girlfriend needs to work their own program. They need to be pursing having an accountability partner or a sponsor/mentor. They need to get themselves into support groups and put security on their devices. If you do not see your partner genuinely pursuing support and care (and solid repentance), you may need to look at whether it is best to continue dating. For a wonderful resource to work through these things, go to purityrestored.com.

What About Sex During Marriage?

Sometimes, those who are not married have questions about sex during marriage. Or they have concerns about what will happen when they get married at some later time. These can be very important conversations. Here are some of the questions we have received:

Are there boundaries for married couples (in terms of purity)?
Yep. Don't do it with someone else other than you spouse. Don't think sexually about anyone other than your spouse. So this would mean no pornography and no fantasizing about anyone other than your spouse. Only include sexual activities that both agree on. Even in the kingdom,

disciples will give and receive differing input on what to include in their bedroom, including masturbatory practices. The list above on "What's Allowed" is what we recommend to couples to figure out any other area that may need to be a boundary. Couples also usually have to work out a number of areas and other healthy boundaries in their sexual relationship such as initiating sex, refusing sex, what level of detail to talk about their sex life with others, how often to have sex, and where and when to have sex. Furthermore, all of these boundaries are reevaluated and restructured if there has been any kind of a betrayal or violation in a marriage or if someone has gotten involved in any kind of pornography or sexual addiction.

If we had a negative sexual experience before, how would we change our perspective about sex? I was sexually abused and in the past, whenever I had sex, my body froze. How would I deal with that in marriage?

Reclaiming the beauty of sex within marriage is often a process for anyone with a negative background in sex. The negative experience might have been sexual abuse as a child, or a negative sexual experience with another adult during the adult years. We encourage any here who are approaching marriage and have had a negative experience to read our book *The Art of Intimate Marriage*. This book provides a more complete answer about the challenges that come up in the marital sexual relationship. You can also read *The Sexual Healing Journey*, which, though from a secular viewpoint and written primarily for married individuals, can also be read for the most part by someone before marriage. Even before you are married, you can receive help in working through any negative experiences you have had sexually. In fact, we would encourage that. Yes, people can come to a positive view of sex; however, that may take relearning about sex as spoken of in chapter one, *What Does the Bible Say about Sex*, or seeing someone professionally.

Is oral sex biblical? When is oral sex OK?

Yes, singles do ask this. In fact, when one of our children had their sex talk, their "how babies are made" talk when they were in first grade, afterwards our child asked me (Jennifer), "Do you put your mouth on daddy's penis?" Dang. Really. Seven! First grade! This was how I answered: "God made our bodies and when you are married, any part of your body can touch any part of their body, and any part of their body can touch any part of yours." Whew! This was a simple explanation to a valid question. I tried to answer honestly without putting any picture in my child's mind. Kids of all ages, and adults as well, have these questions. Is oral sex OK? Once again, as we mention above, we let people decide that for their marriage. We give the What's Allowed list. As far as the question "is it biblical", we would suggest, when you take a look at some of the poetic illusions in Song of Songs, that the answer would be yes.

So when is oral sex OK? In the chapter *Save Yourself,* we address this somewhat for singles. Remember, looking at someone with lust whom you are not married to is sin. Therefore, oral sex with anyone whom you are not married to is definitely well past looking. Enough said.

Is anal sex OK?

This is a question we get asked by both single and married individuals. Before marriage, biblically, anal sex would be sexual immorality and is, therefore, not any more OK than intercourse would be. During marriage, this is something for each couple to make a decision about. Couples do engage in anal sex. This question gets asked at every marriage conference and retreat we speak at. Different leaders and elders in the church may have different answers. We always recommend that couples again use the What's Allowed list to determine the answer for them. However, we always recommend that couples consider the physical consequences of engaging in anal sex. The anus does not have the same kind of flexible tissues as the vagina. The anus also does not secrete lubrication as the vagina does. Anal sex can cause fissures, or cracks, in the walls of the anus. There can be other medical concerns with anal sex that need to be considered.

Finally, this particular sexual practice can be an area of conflict between a husband and wife, and it is vital that spouses remember that demanding or bartering for any sexual practice is contrary to the heart of the sexual relationship in Scripture. Though many husbands request and prefer anal sex, this practice, like any other sexual practice, must be by mutual consent and be of benefit to the relationship in order to fit within the overarching view of sexuality in the Bible.

If I successfully control my sexual desire for a good amount of time, is it possible that I will lose my sexual desire FOREVER (capitals in the original)?

What a real question. If I don't use it, will I lose it? And when we do get married, will the switch just turn back on? This is actually one of the common challenges that newly married couples share. They expected everything to work without any problem and then it didn't quite go that way. They had saved themselves for marriage or they had stopped having sex when they became a Christian. So God will reward us and it'll go really great right? The reality is a little more complicated. Commonly, men do not lack in sexual desire when they do finally get married, though for some couples, it is the wife who has the greater sexual desire and her story may be different about the return of desire.

However, yes, there are some who have controlled their sexual desire response so tightly that they have a challenging time allowing themselves to go ahead and feel the desire and to experience and enjoy sexual feelings. For others, they marry when they are older and the physical drive for sex is lower. Others may find that when they do get married, although they do not think much about sex beforehand (sexual libido/desire), when they do go ahead and engage in sex in a mutually giving and loving way, desire kicks in after they start touching one another. If anything like these scenarios is your story, talk openly about it before marriage and talk about it when you get married in order to have a fulfilling, enjoyable sexual relationship with your spouse. Also, if problems with sexual arousal happen, be open and get help early on. We received some of the best input on our sex life when we were newly married and things weren't going quite as we expected. Be open. Be real. And have fun figuring it all out.

Is it painful to have sex? Do you bleed when you have sex the first time?

Some individuals do have pain when they first have sex. This is true for both men and women. Some men report discomfort of various kinds, and some men who are uncircumcised could potentially experience a tearing of some of the penile tissues, though this is uncommon. For women who have not had sex, there can be some blood due to the tearing of a thin layer of tissue called the hymen that may still be slightly covering the vagina. Some women no longer have that tissue barrier sometimes because their involvement in sports, horseback riding, gymnastics, biking, or other activities already removed the barrier. Many do not experience any pain or bleeding. Though some women do not experience bleeding, they may still have discomfort or pain when the penis enters and during thrusting. This may be due to a woman not getting enough or the right kind of stimulation to build arousal. This can also mean that a woman does not have enough lubrication, either due to lack of arousal, hormonal imbalances, or other medical complications. We tell all couples to take a good lubricant along with them on their honeymoon to help with this. Feel free to ask us a recommendation before you take off on your honeymoon. If someone does continue to experience bleeding, or if the pain continues, they should make sure to seek professional medical help from a sexual medicine specialist.

What is some advice you would give to someone who has never engaged in sex and the fears that come up? And when you do get married, what helped you to get rid of any fears?

Sometimes people do feel fear about how sex is going to go when they are married. The main thing is to start working through that now. You don't have to wait until you're engaged. Start asking the questions and verbalizing the fears you are having. Married brothers and sisters, set a safe atmosphere that allows single brothers and sisters to ask you sensitive questions. Provide a workshop or some teaching, read this book together as a ministry, and then have some open discussions.

When you do get married, talk openly with your spouse about any fears you have. Actually, seek direction on how to have this conversation before you get married and then have it whenever you need after the wedding. At your honeymoon and in those early months of marriage, it will be important that you take whatever time you need to get to know one another's bodies and how to give to one another sexually. Learning to speak openly is usually the number one way to overcome fear and enjoy your sexual relationship.

I have almost no boobs. I look like a 10-year-old girl going through puberty and I'm 22. I'm really afraid my husband will be disappointed/unsatisfied and people always say 'you're beautiful.' I know that but it's also a biological thing.

Both men and women who are not confident about their bodies share that they are concerned how their spouse will respond when they see that body when they get married. For women, there can be a strong awareness that men seem to be very drawn to women's breasts. It is understandable that if you are not well endowed, you might be concerned whether the man you marry will be attracted to your body. And it is true that as a society, we can be very focused on attractiveness and the importance it plays in satisfaction in marriage. However, in a godly marriage, enjoyment of one another's bodies is to be about giving to one another. This does not mean that you should not speak about this concern. If this insecurity creates fear and anxiety, it may be beneficial to talk about it before you get married. We have found that openness has the potential to head off a great number of problems. Do know that after marriage, within the context of a fun and mutually giving sexual relationship, men find their wives breasts incredibly satisfying, whether small or large.

"A loving doe, a graceful deer—may her breasts satisfy you always, may you ever be intoxicated with her love" (Proverbs 5:19). Note that in this scripture, the satisfaction he takes in her breasts is a part of the overall intoxication he feels in connection with her love. Most men will be the first to tell you that the most important thing that makes them happy in their marriage and sexual relationship is how their wife makes them feel. Our guess is that if you marry someone who is dedicated to God, this will be your experience as well.

Why do the marrieds not speak of sexual intimacy when a single is in the group? (Hush the conversation, make gestures to one another that they will continue talking when the 'single' left or another day)?
AND
How can we change the non-dialogue within our church? Why can't we educate singles, dating or not, what to expect in marriage so that we don't romanticize it and remain unprepared?

We hope the married among us, including the ones writing this book, hear the appeal in these questions. Married women, your single sisters want to talk to you. You might feel like you don't know all of the answers but you can grow together in finding them. You may feel like you can't help guide a single sister when it's not going well in your own marriage. Let this spur you on to getting help in your marriage. Then, with wisdom, share what you learn with your single sister. Married men, your single brothers want to talk to you. You could feel that if your own struggles aren't going well, you have nothing to offer them. Married brothers and sisters, open up your homes and your hearts and let the single, campus, and teens in. Seek input on how to respond if you're not sure, but let them know it's OK to talk about it. And don't wait for them to ask. Ask permission from them to initiate the conversation. "Hey, I was wondering how this is going for you and if you have any questions. Is it OK if we talk about this?"

Sex and the Older Single

"Can you address sexuality and the older single woman in her 50s and 60s and beyond?" and "I will be 70 years old soon and am not married. The church seems to coach the younger sisters. I am still desirable and desiring. What about me?"

There is a general myth out there that older people either are not having sex, are not interested in sex, or don't have sexual feelings and desires. This can be especially true for older women. As Ray Romano in Everybody Loves Raymond says to his studio parents about their sex life, "Aren't you tired?" Though you may be an older male or female, you may still have the desire for orgasm and a sexual relationship. You may still be challenged by pornography and masturbation and the pull toward extramarital sex. Others among you may feel quite differently and are perfectly happy not to be bothered by it. Ultimately, most of this book is just as addressed to you as it is to any younger single reading this.

However, there are some unique challenges for you. People make the assumptions we mentioned above and you may have to be the one educating them about the fallacy of those assumptions. Also, you may have had many different sexual relationships through the years. You could be carrying a number of feelings, hurts, and traumas. And perhaps you have secretly felt that your sexual past is no longer relevant. It is relevant. Be open with someone. Your process of healing may also end up helping many others. You may also be an older single who is struggling with some serious levels of use of pornography and other sexual outlets, and the patterns might be long standing or, with the advent of the Internet, they may have peaked in the last few years. And those involved in your life, because of their assumption that older people aren't interested in sex, may not even think to ask you about this area. Starting the conversation may be up to your convictions. Do not let shame, guilt, or pride keep you from getting the help you need.

Can you "fully" know God if you live a celibate life and are a single disciple your entire life?

That's a fair question. We have reviewed that sexuality is a language between us and God in order to know God more fully, and that can be equally true for someone who engages sexually and someone who does not. However, let's take a further look at the words of Paul about this. "I wish that all men were even as I myself" (1 Cor 7:7). Then again he says, "It is good for them to stay unmarried" (v. 8). And then he gives a clincher. "Those who marry will face many troubles in this life, and I want to spare you this." Dang, not much of an endorsement for marriage. Why does he say all this? He makes it clear later when he says,

> "I would like you to be free from concern. An unmarried man is concerned about the Lord's affairs—how he can please the Lord. But a married man is concerned about the affairs of this world—how he can please his wife—and his interests are divided. An unmarried woman or virgin is concerned about the Lord's affairs: Her aim is to be devoted to the Lord in both body and spirit. But a married woman is concerned about the affairs of this world—how she can please her husband. I am saying this for your won good ... that you may live in a right way in undivided devotion to the Lord."
>
> 1 Corinthians 7:32-35

The word for concern in this passage is *merimnao* which means anxious, distracted, drawn in opposite directions and divided into parts. The word for devoted here is *euprosedros*, which means constantly attending to. Paul here is saying that a married man or woman who is supposed to be devoted to pleasing a spouse, including sexually, is pulled in opposite directions and that there is great benefit to someone's service and relationship with God when their devotion does not have to be divided in that way.

Jesus said, "The one who sent me is with me; he has not left me alone, for I always do what pleases him" (John 8:29). What an incredibly clear mandate for the importance of being with God. Jesus says God is with Him. That God has not left Him alone. You see Jesus' every action was motivated by the desire to please God. As a church, we often hold up marriage and sexuality in marriage as if they are the *sin qua non*, the absolute peak of how we can live in Christ. In fact, there may sometimes be a basic inhospitableness toward single people in church and within the church, we can fail to grasp the important role of celibacy. It is important that we carefully examine what Scripture has to say about these things. Jesus himself held up the example of "those who live like eunuchs for the sake of the kingdom of heaven" (Matt 19:12) and Jesus Himself was celibate. As a family of God, we need to honor celibacy rather than make it sound like some kind of illness.

It is not about whether it is better to be married or better to be single. It is not about weighing the different benefits of celibacy versus what is gained through sex. In both states, we can be in communion with God, knowing Him deeply in uniquely wonderful ways. Someone who is celibate and single their entire life has the unique situation of never being distracted by a partner; never being divided from their devoted knowing of God. God speaks through His physical creation, and yes that includes sex. But knowing God is also far greater than the physical creation as well. "This is eternal life, that you may know God" (John 10:17). That knowledge of God begins here on this earth, in whatever state we are in, and continues for eternity. We must all, no matter our sexual lives, be devoted to our knowledge of God.

Remember these two scriptures:

Proverbs 2:2: "My son, if you accept my words … turning your ear to wisdom and applying your heart to understanding … if you look for it as for silver and search for it as for hidden treasure, then you will understand the fear of the Lord and find the knowledge of God" (emphasis added).

Jeremiah 9:24: "Let him who boasts boast about this: that he - (yada) me, that I am the Lord who exercises kindness, justice and righteousness on earth, for in these I delight" (emphasis and parenthetical added).

So, whatever your state, whether in a sexual relationship or not, let us all be devoted to our knowledge of God.

For those of you with similar questions, our prayer for you is that you will pursue sexual purity—not only when you are single, but also when you are married. As you do this, you will bring God glory by how you live your life here with your eyes focused on heaven.

CHAPTER 14

WHAT'S A TEEN TO DO?

You are in your teen years and somehow you ended up with this book in your hands. However you have come to this point—kicking and screaming or relieved and intrigued—congratulations on seeking out biblical and factual information about sexuality. You may still have questions, concerns and anxiety about this topic. Let's listen to what some other teens have to say, and then figure out how to live out God's calling in your generation.

We have raised four teenagers. In the midst of teaching about sex to teens and singles, we have realized that we have made our own mistakes in how we have talked about sex during these years. We'd like to explore with you what you as a teen are experiencing. Some of these may be your circumstances:

- Almost all your friends (especially those outside of the church) have boyfriends or girlfriends.
- Your classmates or sports team members talk openly about the sex they are having.
- Your friends have asked you if you're gay because they have not seen you with someone.

- In almost every show you watch, people are sexually active, including teenagers.
- Your parents are not comfortable talking about sex. In fact it is really awkward. And you really have no interest in talking with them about it.
- You have feelings of attraction to someone of the same gender, to both genders, to no one, or you are not sure if you are the right gender, and you don't feel like you have anyone you can talk to.
- You notice one or both of your parents seem to struggle with touch. You wonder if they even have sex.
- You suspect that one or both of your parents have had sex with someone outside of their marriage.
- You feel like the rules at church about what teenage boys and girls can or cannot do together are rigid and the rules about modesty for girls are outdated and guy-focused.

These may be some of your situations. So we began to wonder, *What are other teens going through and what are they thinking about sex?* Actually, in 2012, someone did a research study of teens in America (this was a general audience and not limited to Christian teens) and we'd like to share the results.[1] See if any of this reflects what it is like for you:

- 46% of teens say that parents most influence their decisions about sex. By comparison, just 20% say friends most influence their decisions.
- Eight in ten teens (80%) say that it would be much easier for teens to delay sexual activity and avoid teen pregnancy if they were able to have more open, honest conversations about these topics with their parents.
- Six in ten teens (62%) wish they were able to talk more openly about relationships with their parents.

---

[1] "With One Voice" at thenationalcampaign.org

- Most teens (65% of girls and 57% of boys) who have had sex say they wish they had waited.
- A significant percentage of teens (63%) and adults (72%) agree that "teen boys often receive the message that they are expected to have sex."
- Most teens (71%) and adults (77%) also agree that "teen girls often receive the message that attracting boys and looking sexy is one of the most important things they can do."
- Most teens (93% of girls and 88% of boys) say they would rather have a boyfriend/girlfriend and not have sex rather than have sex but not have a boyfriend or girlfriend.
- Most teens (71%) and adults (81%) agree that sharing nude or semi-nude images of themselves or other teens electronically (through cell phones, websites, and/or social media networks) leads to more sex in real life.
- 85% of teens agreed that parents believe they should talk to their kids about sex but often don't know what to say, how to say it, or when to start.

As a teen, you might be more open to talking about sexuality if it were done in a real and authentic way. It would help if adults took the responsibility to be non-shaming, gracious, and open; to provide real conversations and not lectures. Regardless, you know your parents' experience was different than yours and that there are unique things happening in your world in the area of sexuality. Our own adult kids tell us that we have no idea what things were really like for them. So instead of us telling you what we think your world is like and how to navigate it, we thought we'd get the words of those who have been living in it. We decided to talk to young men and women who are committed Christians about their experiences in high school in the area of sexuality. We asked what they had seen, heard, or had been told. They also told us where they heard it—in high school, from their friends, at home, at church, and on TV, movies, social media, and the Internet. Here are their exact words:

AT SCHOOL

In school, I had more friends that were sexually active than those who weren't. And they would tell me their stories and they would be specific on what they did and they would be proud too. In the back of my head I knew I shouldn't be hanging out with them, hearing what they did, but I still hung out with them because it was a taste of what's out there. It made me struggle, I'm not gonna lie. But I never got open about my struggle when it came to hearing about people having sex.

My school was definitely surrounded by sexual activity and partying. It got to the point where they put up a sign that said "no latex" and we figured that was no condoms at school. It was definitely everywhere at school. You couldn't go to class and not hear a story or have someone show you a video they saw or hear someone say, "Hey, check out that girl." It was a battlefield at school, but I never confessed about the temptation when I heard that kind of stuff. It made it difficult to live a pure life.

* * * * *

At high school among my friends, I knew people were having sex. It seemed a very nonchalant kind of thing. It wasn't talked about, but everyone knew it was going on. No type of monogamous thing. Very casual.

* * * * *

In high school, definitely as a young man, the goal of many young men was to have sex, so I would hear a lot about that with guys who ended up hooking up with a girl or had a girlfriend and they would usually tell stories about the most recent escapade. I heard a lot of personal sexual experiences from people. Being on a sports team I heard a lot of that and it became synonymous with how masculine you were; how much sex you had and how much opportunity you had.

☆ ☆ ☆ ☆ ☆

Definitely I had friends who were sexually active whether that was with girlfriends or they were hooking up and would go to a party. That was happening a lot in high school. I would hear stories from other guys about what they were doing with other girls. Guys would send pictures. People sent nude photos of each other. One time I was in one conversation waiting for basketball practice and one of the guys walked into the gym and everybody knew that he'd hooked up at a party with some girl and everybody rushed to him and asked what happened. I didn't have any experience. My experience came from what I heard and that experience was what I believed what sex is.

I heard a lot from people often. It was mostly with one crowd of people, the popular kids, going to the parties and hanging out. It was not everyone, but it was a good number of people that I was hearing it from. And pornography was a big deal.

☆ ☆ ☆ ☆ ☆

I felt insecure in high school because I wasn't active as some of the other kids were. It almost seemed like they were much cooler, much more respected, much more popular. It's like if you didn't know about it, then you weren't as accepted in the circles. I felt super insecure. I heard them, but I didn't know what they were saying or talking about. You almost feel like sex becomes more important than someone's personality or character, etc. when you're looking for women to date. It's like what's lifted up in conversations and pornography, and you want to find a girl that looks like this and can do this.

* * * * *

At school, sexuality was definitely encouraged. I had a lot of friends that all dated each other so everyone slept with everyone. To give your body over to boys was the thing to do and I would say very much encouraged at parties. There were a lot of parties, and it was encouraged there when people were intoxicated. An overly sexualized environment, where everyone was with everyone.

* * * * *

On my basketball team, it was everyone for their own and you did what you wanted. I had three lesbians on my team my freshman year. They were the odd man out at school; probably the only three lesbians at school. That influenced me at school, like saying it was wrong to be a lesbian because you were alienated from everyone else. Lesbians played basketball and baseball at school. I think what I heard at home regarding sexuality and homosexuality was that it was not encouraged. It was gross and that we just didn't do that. These were the things I saw and the messages I got, which had an effect on how I lived out being a lesbian in high school.

* * * * *

In middle school, I was friends with someone and what shocked me the most was this girl had Facetimed a guy naked and they egged each other on to do inappropriate things. It was unexpected at middle school age because I'd kept myself pretty sheltered. On my lacrosse team, there were girls who talked about having sex sometimes and going to parties. I thought, "Why would you want to do that?" And then, the first time one of my friends brought it up was sophomore year and she had just told me that she gave a friend's older brother a blowjob in their living room. That was surprising to me because I thought it was gross. But then when, that book called Burn Book, when that app was a big deal, a lot was discussed about people. Not so much about sex, but different types of jobs and were they good or not. It was talked on the Burn Book a lot.

* * * * *

In high school, there was a lot about what you wear, what the girls were wearing in order to catch the eyes of guys in school. That was not how I was raised but it's the way our culture conditioned us. That that is how sex is. It is something that you give away freely. Like something my older brother told me. I was dating someone for about a month. My brother said, "Wait until you date a month before you have sex with him." I was so surprised he said that. I was sheltered because most of my friends were disciples. That opened my eyes like, "Wow, this is normal." A lot of my friends started having sex in 8th grade. It wasn't necessarily about love or like knowing who you are. It was more like, "Oh, it's fun" and "Everyone's doing it."

* * * * *

There was a lot of shame in my house about sex, but it wasn't that way with my friend's at school at all. They were super open talking about sex. Somebody would have sex with someone, and then they were having it with anyone. From kissing, and then hooking up, to having sex. You do one thing with one

219

person then all your morals go out the window, which is what I saw with a lot of my friends.

* * * * *

At school, as far as our teachers, what stuck out and I will never forget, my health teacher told us that masturbation is the only way to stay abstinent. She would say that you should stay abstinent and you shouldn't do anything until you're married and have a child. I really disagreed about that. That was the first time I talked to my mom. We were taught masturbation was wrong. That was the only time I talked about anything sexual before I became a disciple.

* * * * *

My friends at school. All of them were having sex. A lot of times it would happen pretty soon after they started dating someone. It was like wild. It would happen in cars, in their back yard. You didn't want to get caught by your parents. That was the biggest thing. I saw a lot of my friends get really hurt because of it. They cried a lot because of it.

I think the biggest thing is like when I wasn't a disciple I was constantly torn between wanting to have sex, because all of my friends were, and with God not wanting that for me.

* * * * *

One of my friends during freshman year, I remember very specifically his sharing he'd had sex with a girl. I remember that very specifically. In our area, you get a girlfriend and you have sex. So they'd have some kind of sex after they hooked up and they'd develop a tight relationship. And then the guys would be overwhelming with how clingy they were and the girls would break up with them.

* * * * *

At school, it was mostly coarse joking and stuff. The talking about it was explicit and there were no boundaries around it. And then sometimes I would go to some parties I would see people hooking up and disappear and wasn't sure what was happening beyond that.

At Home

At home, it was harder to live a pure life at home especially whenever I hung out with my older brother or his friends. One time at a party, I wanted to get time with my brother, but then he started to talk about his experience of having sex and all these girls he had sex with and how he had a girlfriend but he would still cheat on her. I didn't find that right, but I wasn't speaking out, "I don't think that's right. Why would you do that? Have you told her?" I didn't have the strength to confront my brother about it. So I kept it to myself. I wasn't confessing temptation, "I heard this. It's in my thoughts." So again, it made it hard to live a pure life at home. With my dad, the brothers challenged me once to have him help me block my computer from pornography. I asked him for help and he said, "That's OK. You're at that age." That didn't help at all. At home, I didn't have any support.

* * * * *

At home, it was never talked about unless I brought it up. But it was still not talked about very much. I remember my parents talking about it a couple times growing up, but there was never

any open dialogue about it. Any explanation like what it is anatomically or emotionally.

* * * * *

With my family, if I had pursued asking about it they would have
talked about it with me. But it was like, that is not something
we talk about openly. We need to be in a confined confidential
room and be careful who hears. The culture of "Let's not talk
about it." In my situation, when I was giving into sexual temptation and exploring sexuality, you know the consequence of your
actions and it's scary to talk about it and you don't talk about
it especially with Christian parents who live the Christian life.
You feel intimidated. I wish my parents would have brought it
up more. Even one of my parents fell into sin with someone in
the church and I only learned that after I fell into sin and I wish
I'd learned that earlier. I would have like to have talked about it
earlier.

I don't think I even got an official talk with my parents. If
they did it wasn't very impacting. My parents were open. but
conservative and this is a liberal touchy subject and they don't
talk about it much other than in a conventional atmosphere.

* * * * *

With my parents, I can remember two sex talks. One was when I
was younger and I asked, "Where do babies come from" and my
mom gave me the stork example. When I was about 15 or 16, I
had a conversation with my dad and he talked about, "Do you
know what sex is?" "I think so." It was awkward. "Do you like
anybody?" I was super hesitant in that conversation. He asked a
lot of questions to draw me out and see what I knew. But I was

ashamed and scared to talk about it so that I never came back to that conversation.

And then I had many family members who made comments. When I hit puberty, I had a strong growth spurt at 16, and my family, my aunts and uncles, I remember them making jokes about getting an STD. Making jokes about using a condom. I got that often. As someone who had no experience, I didn't know how a condom worked. I would awkwardly laugh it off or brush it off.

* * * * *

One time, my sibling and I walked in on a family member watching pornography and we hadn't seen it before. We were watching it and he saw us and freaked out and it caused this huge commotion. And my parents and grandparents got into it and there was a huge fight. We were like "What was that?" And that sparked my curiosity.

* * * * *

What I saw at home, well … we didn't talk much about sexuality. My mom and dad I think tried to have a conversation with me maybe at 16, but it wasn't impacting enough for me to remember it. We didn't talk about sexuality much in our house.

* * * * *

My mom never really talked to me about it. She gave me a sex talk, the natural talk, how sex is natural. It was always talked about that it's not going to be until marriage. I always had it in my mind it was for marriage and not something you do in high school. But it was never really talked about.

* * * * *

My parents never talked to me about sex ever, but the experience I had from it was when one of my parents committed adultery. And yet it still wasn't talked about in my house. I definitely heard that you don't do it until you're married. You'd better be a disciple. But we didn't talk about it too much.

* * * * *

What made it even more taboo was when one of my parent's partners brought a lot of pornography into the house. So it was something that was happening, but it wasn't talked about. There was a lot of shame in the house.

* * * * *

I didn't feel safe about talking about it. We had this talk one time. My mom asked me if I'd had sex, but it wasn't an environment I felt safe in. I got super defensive.

At Church

At church, it was easier. I definitely feel safe. I feel the confidence to talk about my temptation. I knew I had the support. I just felt safe with the body. I knew I had people who had the same mindset and the same goal. So it was easier to be open with a brother once I saw him. "Hey, I did this. I did that." And they would ask me, "Were you alone? What triggered you?" So I would try to hang out with the brothers rather than stay at home. I always wanted to go to events and go hang out and that was because I just knew there was something better. There was something about wanting to please God that felt better than wanting to please my desires.

* * * * *

Nobody talked about it at church. Ever. Unless it was "Don't do it" and "Don't think about it." It wasn't talked about at all. It was not explained or discussed in a way that made it ok to bring it up. But it was "When you're married it's great" at the end of the conversation.

* * * * *

At church, it was definitely more hush-hush. You didn't mention sex because it was viewed as so wrong. It was the culture. Since we're young and not married it was wrong to talk about it, not just about a lustful way, but about anything else. That you have to be careful because you don't want to cause somebody to struggle.

Even with teens that weren't disciples, there were teens that would talk about a sexual escapade or adventure. This was in late middle school and early high school. They came to the teens because their parents were disciples. At sleepovers and hangouts, when they felt more safe, they would talk about that stuff. So it was not as much as at school, but it was there.

* * * * *

I think growing up in the church, I was definitely taught to wait until you're married and this is what the Bible says about sex and I felt aware of that even in high school. But there is defi-nitely like a strong curiosity especially when you hear about it a lot at school or even amongst other teens who were sexually active. I knew kids in my ministry that were having sex. And you know, we loved our ministry and loved being with each other, but there was this, "I have this life here and then I have this other life where I can be what I want and do what I want."

* * * * *

I heard a lot about sexuality at church. Starting about 8th grade into freshman year. It was impacting how I saw sexuality. I went to a private Lutheran school, and even if you had spiritual values and morals, that didn't matter because everyone was hooking up in the bleachers at school even though it was a private Christian school and purity was encouraged. I heard a lot of stories about how people would do sexual things on campus and in the bathroom; wherever they could. That influenced me a lot in how I saw sexuality in regards to religion. At church, in high school, there were a lot of girls who went to church who got pregnant. Purity was not revered.

* * * * *

At church when I was a teen we didn't talk about it at all.

* * * * *

At church, it was shocking to hear about Christian teens who had left God and then were having sex. Or people who were studying the Bible who were falling into that type of sin. When you're in the church you're definitely not protected.

But teens are not just in the sexual society. Not everything is sinful. We still have fun hanging out. Not everything is sexual, totally surrounded. But everything is so accessible. It's ok to be curious, but it's possible to not be sexual.

*****

At a church conference, they talked about the boundaries God wants for sex. And the speed our bodies go about it is not the speed God wants. That kissing is outside of the "what God wants" in the realm of sex because it speeds things up so quickly. I thought that made sense because a lot of my boyfriends would ask as soon as we started kissing, "Hey, do you wanna have sex?" The body goes from 0 to 100 so fast.

IN THE MEDIA (TV, MOVIES, INTERNET, SOCIAL MEDIA)

In the media, there is definitely a lot of women who are half nude. So, it was hard. At home, whenever I wanted to watch a show, either they would mention something about sex or they would show something that would trigger that temptation of wanting to see even more. Again, I knew that was just a taste of what's in the world.

*****

I knew it wasn't as it is portrayed on TV and movies, but it was portrayed as everybody is doing it and you need to do it to be happy. It was like very intense and you can't control yourself. The build-up was very intense. Not this natural thing that happened between people, but more like people couldn't control themselves anymore. And it was always portrayed between people that were hyper-attractive and very young. Those are the people that get to do it and other people don't get to because they are not as attractive.

*****

In TV and movies, as far as extramarital, premarital, any sex like that, it is portrayed as a thrill and sex with a stable married partner is looked down on. The husband always wants to get something and the wife doesn't want to give him sex and the husband makes a lot of stupid mistakes.

* * * * *

If I was watching movies my parents were on top of sex scenes, making us look away and fast forward. My parents were really good about what we were watching. Even at home and other people's houses. With the internet, you almost feel like sex becomes more important than someone's personality or character etc. You're looking for women to date and like what's lifted up in those conversations and in pornography is that you want to find a girl that looks like this and can do this and they don't have worth. You build up that mentality and then, even after you begin battling it and you know it's not important, you realize you keep thinking that way and ask yourself, "Why am I still concerned about it?"

* * * * *

I grew up watching ACE Ventura, Austin Powers, and Dumb and Dumber. A lot of sexual innuendos. We weren't allowed to watch movies with sexual content in it, but we watched a lot of movies with sexual innuendos, and we rode the road about what is appropriate and allowed.

* * * * *

With movies, we watched movies at my friend's house and they weren't parent-approved movies. Pornography? I was exposed to it at 10 or 12 I think. In middle school, there were some kids talking about websites and stuff like that. And on phones and social media, they subtly promote things and the sinful nature craves it. And it won't get old and the craving will always be there, like on social media and Snapchat.

* * * * *

Social media definitely wasn't good. It's hard in our generation because masturbation and pornography are starting to become good. There's a lot of things on the Internet saying it's healthy to masturbate and to be sexually active. Things that were never talked about were suddenly popular. What surprised me the most was that it was all girls talking about it. And social media, like Instagram, it's hard to control what comes up on your feed. A lot of things are pretty sexual on Instagram. Snapchat too is dangerous because you can pretty quickly send a picture.

TV shows, they are very graphic. There was a show I watched. I was sheltered and skipped all of it, but you could tell a scene was coming because of the build-up to the scene was really graphic. And you'd always see people in bras and under-wear making out.

* * * * *

When it comes to TV and movies, it did influence how I wanted to dress and how I carried myself around men. It was like that's what you had to do to be loved by a man.

ADVICE AND WORDS OF WISDOM FROM THE TRENCHES

I did get open about what I was seeing on TV because that is a common thing to see and it was relatable to other brothers because we all watched entertainment. So it was easier to get open. Because a brother can give you advice or guide you to a scripture, but it is your effort that depends on whether you are going to deny your flesh.

* * * * *

There have been a few times the teen leader would separate boys and girls and talk about our purity. I think it would have helped if there were more. That way we can ask more questions. Because when you hear those lessons you start thinking, What could I do different? What do I do to avoid this situation? How do I find the courage to say this? That way we don't get a hint of temptation.

* * * * *

Tell parents to have the conversation even if it's a little bit awkward. Starting in 6th grade you're thinking about it and it's on your mind. So it's not like your parents would be initiating all this new stuff with you.

* * * * *

For a lot of people sex is the end goal and then a relationship ends up miserable because they don't understand that a relationship doesn't have substance. Sex is ultimately it. A lot of the teens, they get confused after their relationships deteriorate after they had sex. The guys seemed more damaged than the girls. It's hard living in a world that promotes that so much.

* * * * *

I had a few mentors while I was in high school that had some
conversations with me, asking me if I was having sex and sharing
their experience about why it's good to wait and what the Bible
says about it.

So What's a Teen to Do?

In these thoughts from teens there is much wisdom to be found. We'd
like to share what we noticed.

As a teen, you aren't thinking about sex all the time. You enjoy just
hanging out. It is also really clear that there are a lot of people around
you having sex. A lot of you are hearing about it from those you hang
out with at school, in sports, and also at church. It sounds like many
of you wish you could talk with someone about how much of a pull sex
presents. You wish it was talked about more often and more openly at
church and at home. It would help if you had a mentor to talk to about
the explicit stories you are hearing and also about relationships overall.
Teens, it is also obvious that you might have a number of questions, feelings, and thoughts, but that it is uncomfortable talking about these. For
parents who are reading this, it is our responsibility to make it easier for
our teens to talk about sex, not just when they engage in something that
concerns you. And, parents, when you make bad choices sexually, some
open, real, genuine sharing could go a long way toward helping your teen
feel like they could open up.

It was great hearing from a few young men who felt like they had
someone to talk to. However, one of your biggest needs might be some
help finding a mentor, someone other than your parent to talk to. It
sounds like you'd like your parents to talk openly with you, but that
sometimes you'd like to be able to talk with someone other than your
parent. If your ministry is not actively helping make that happen, you
may need to be the one to speak up in order to make that happen.

It also seems like you're hearing a lot of conflicting opinions about
whether engaging sexually is really as wrong as your parents or church

state. We recommend you take some serious time to examine the chapter *Save Yourself.* The best way to answer that question is to dig into Scripture. You need to be prepared with intelligent, biblical answers, not just for others, but for your own doubts and questions. Even if you are wrestling to find your own faith, the Scriptures do a good job of lifting the fog.

Teens, from what you shared, it would be a good idea to pay attention to what you are watching, listening to, and reading. If you have the desire to figure out God's plan for sexuality, you may need to take a serious look at your social media use, your social life (who you're hanging out with), the shows and movies you watch, and the apps you use; not just those that are explicitly sexual but those that tell sexual jokes.

You may relate to the teens who talked about all the sensuality around them being arousing sexually. If this is your experience, this sensitive topic may be difficult to share because you fear how people will react. The young woman who shared about having homosexual attractions was surrounded by reactions that definitely didn't make her feel like she could talk freely. You may be able to relate. You might struggle with other attractions that are hard to talk about. There is a forum for teens on the Strength in Weakness website that we recommend. Guy Hammond has a link on his website to set up some time to talk with him or with one of the young men or women in the Strength in Weakness ministry who provide support. Take advantage of it.

Perhaps you are one of those who feels insecure with and doesn't always understand sexual comments people make. We hope you have gotten some good information in this book that might answer some of those questions. However, if you have some other questions and feel like you're not sure where to turn, we'd love to hear from you. Drop us a line at tjkonzen@yahoo.com or jenniferkonzen@yahoo.com.

You might feel a war raging inside of you—wanting to try out sexual impulses but also wanting to follow God. Sometimes, the people you should be able to trust, or who should be your role models, haven't been setting the best example. Your own parents may not be choosing well.

The person who studied the Bible with you or someone you look up to in your ministry may fall into sexual sin. In order to fight this battle, you may need some solid armor. There is a phrase in certain translations of the Bible you may find helpful; the phrase "gird yourselves." In 1 Peter 1:13, the literal meaning of what you are called to do is to "gird up the loins of your mind"; to put secure clothing or armor around the parts of your bodies (or minds, or hearts) that are vulnerable in order to protect them from harm. To be obedient children to God, to keep from conforming to sinful desires to satisfy the flesh, you may need to do some serious girding. Ground yourself deeply in the Word and you'll be better able to withstand the pressure of what your peers do and say. Remember, "Do not let anyone look down on you because you are young, but set an example for the believers in speech, in conduct, in love, in faith and in purity" (1 Timothy 4:12).

We are rooting for you. So are all the witnesses in heaven, and so are your brothers and sisters in the faith throughout the world. You have the opportunity to set an example and call the family of God higher. We honor you and we fight beside you.

SECTION FIVE

PARENTING AND SEXUALITY

CHAPTER 15

THE TALK: HOW TO TALK
TO YOUR KIDS ABOUT SEX

Just seeing the title of this chapter makes some parents quail. Having "the talk" can bring up an amazing amount of anxiety for parents. You may feel very strongly that you want your kids to come to you with any questions they have, but you have always felt incredibly uncomfortable talking about sex. You don't like talking about it with your spouse or anyone else, for that matter. Or maybe you explained how babies are made when your child was younger, but you're not sure how to talk during the middle school and teenage years. So where do you start?

First Things First

It is crucial for parents who want to lead their children in making good choices sexually to remember the most important thing: First and foremost, how is your relationship with God? How is your walk with Him? How are you doing as a parent in your own knowledge and intimacy with God? This is the most important part of parenting your children, especially in the area of sexuality. Prioritize your relationship with God above all else. Steep yourself in knowing Him. When you do, He will direct your footsteps, even in this very sensitive area of parenting. In trying to figure out how to teach your children about sex, another area to check is your own view of sexuality. This is strongly affected by how you were raised. How did your parents convey information about what happens during puberty or how babies were made? I (Tim) have a vivid memory of my brother, sister, and I being called by our dad to come sit at the dinner table for an important discussion. We assumed he was going to share about something like a new job or who he was going to marry (my parents divorced when I was young). I remember sitting there with all our hands carefully folded, wondering. But all our assumptions were wrong. He proceeded to talk about drugs and sex to all three of us together. I think I've blocked a good part of that conversation out of my brain.

How was your talk? Did you have one? Many adults have no memory of a talk, or the memory they have is a bit traumatic. Or they had the talk but the subject was never broached again. How did that affect your own feelings about sexuality? It's also important to be aware of other things you experienced that may influence how you view sex. Explore chapter one and two before having this talk with your child. Being aware of your own experience can help guide how you speak with your children. God's beautiful plan for sexuality will be your anchor.

How would you rate yourself on your personal understanding of God's plan for sex? How is your own life going sexually? How well are you following that plan? Do you struggle with pornography? Do you battle lust? Do you talk to the brothers or sisters about any sexual sins in your life, including any ways that you have struggled in the past or are struggling currently?

One of the best ways that you can guide your children in the sexual choices they make throughout life is by making sure you are personally following the sexual ethic as it is laid out in God's Word. Check your convictions, repent in any area you need to repent in, get help, and get in the Word, strengthening your understanding of what the Scriptures say about sex.

For those of you who are married, if you are having issues in your own marital sexual relationship, get some help and guidance. The best "talk" you can have with your children is by setting an example within your marriage of how to live out the marital sexual relationship. For those of you who have been married in the past but are single now, there may be some challenges you had in your past sexual relationships. Talk with someone about those things. You may be wondering by this point, Why should we do these things and have these conversations? Because if sexuality has been problematic in your marital sexual relationships (whether present or past), this will affect how you speak with your kids about sex. If you have questions, get them answered. Go through the chapter on God's view of sexuality and deepen your own convictions. Before you speak with your children, grow in your own understanding of what the Scriptures say and change the things in your own life to reflect what you see in the Bible.

What Are You Going to Name It?

No, not what are you going to name your child. This is the age-old question of what you are going to name *it*. *It* being that part of your child's body that many are uncomfortable calling by its given name. That would be the penis, the vulva and vagina, the breasts, or the scrotum. When parents speak with their young children, it is very common for them to use euphemisms for sexual body parts. In the Western world, some common terms for the penis and vagina have been wee wee, pee pee, teetee, wawa, birdie, bits, area, and privates. The vagina has been called pootie, cookie, foofoo, hoohoo, popo, cooter/coochie, mucker, peach, girly bits, front bum, flower, fanny, and various female names like Mary, Susie, or Minnie. Breasts have been called num nums, cha chas, ta tas, boobs/boobies, and tee tees. The penis has been called a weenis, ding-a-ling, winky, hotdog, tinkle, willy, weiner, dooney, guy stuff, and peter. The scrotum and testicles have been called nuts, jewels, the boys, balls, knackers, rocks, gear, and cojones. Other cultures and languages of the world use many other terms. You name it, it's probably been used and you may have a few to add to this list.

Though reading some of these can cause laughter, it is important to realize that calling a child's penis and vagina the correct names has a much better chance of taking away any mysterious stigma that using nicknames can cause. Using the correct names sets a foundation for talking openly and honestly about sexual topics and the body. We do not use nicknames for the other parts of our body (well OK, the nose has a few), and the primary reason we use them for the sexual parts is due to our own discomfort. Using correct terms can help a child develop and understand that just like their elbow, their pinky finger, and their cheek, their sexual parts are just other parts of their body, all of which are special and made by God. Giving these parts their normal names says that they are normal and it is good to talk about them.

We have four children. Three of them are boys. When they were young, I (Jennifer) would take them all out to do some errands. I began to notice that when we passed the lingerie section of a major department store, like JC Penney or Macy's, my boys would look away, laugh, fidget, or make a joke. So we talked lightly about it, how both boys and girls have to wear underwear and that girls also wear bras. That sent them into a whole other level of hilarity and discomfort. So when we arrived home, we ended up dancing all together around the house, throwing out our hands and shouting, "Bras! Underwear! Bras! Underwear!" They all still joke about that. These items are merely pieces of clothing, but we are not always sure what to do with our eyes and thoughts. It is important that we make it normal to talk about these kinds of things. This is very much the approach we encourage for parents. Call sexual things their correct names. Making their own anatomy normal and natural is one of the many good gifts you can give your children.

Touch in the Family

Parents often have questions about what kind of touching and affection should occur in the family—between siblings, between parents and their children, and between the parents. Ask yourself, Am I affectionate with my child? Do I feel any constraints about being affectionate, either due to their age or their gender? Also, parents often wonder if their children should see them touch one another in any intimate way (i.e., touches to the buttocks or kissing). Let's examine these things.

A parent in one of our workshops asked, "As a parent, is it appropriate for my son or daughter to lay their head on my lap or my thigh? Should there be a pillow in between?" What a genuine question. Some of us have experienced sexual abuse or violating sexual touches, and we may fear these things happening to our children. Also, as our children are going through puberty and coming into adolescence, they become more aware of their own bodies and of sex; we may wonder how to navigate touch in a way that is both loving and wise.

In general, healthy affection in the family is an important part of healthy sexual development. The lack of physical affection can send a number of negative messages or cause a child to wonder what is wrong with them. Women talk about the fun in their relationship with their father when they were little, and the switch that seemed to go off as they entered puberty and the teen years. Men tell about little or no affection within their family and the lack of expression of both physical and verbal affection as they were growing up. Those young boys weren't sure what was wrong, but the message they got was that there was something unlikable about them. Many adults, as they look back at their childhood, talk about the pain of not being touched or held by their parent(s). Touch can be a touchy topic (pun intended) because violating touch can be traumatizing. However, a lack of warm touch can convey some serious and important messages that parents need to be aware of.

As mentioned in a previous chapter, when families have rigid, perhaps unconscious rules about touch in order to keep touch from becoming sexual, this can lead to problems with sexuality and can once again convey that topics about sexuality and the body are off limits. As families, let us find how we can imitate God in how He holds us in His hands, gathers us under His arms, enfolds us in His wings, and carries us close to His heart. God is a God who communicates His love to us through affectionate terms. Let us imitate His heart of affection in our marriage and with our children.

Normative Sexual Exploration

In an earlier chapter, we covered what kind of sexual behaviors are considered normative, or normal, for a child to engage in as they grow. See chapter four, The Development of Sexuality, if you have not done that yet. We are going to review a few of those things here. Parents are often concerned and worried when they see their young child engaging in behaviors that seem sexual. It is important that parents know that many of the behaviors, though perhaps disturbing for the parent, are normal exploration during child development. This includes self-exploration and mutual sexual and genital exploration. Children touch themselves. Girls might put their fingers into their vagina and touch their vulva. Boys might fondle their penis and scrotum. They often touch one another's genitals, either with their hands or sometimes with their mouths. Though all of these exploring behaviors can be considered typical, typical does not mean that they go unaddressed. Children may sometimes simulate sexual behaviors. Though these kinds of behaviors are not a definite indication of sexual abuse, a careful exploration by drawing the child out would be important. As you do that, remember, children may have a hard time saying they don't like something or that it made them feel uncomfortable. This can be an important time to teach children how to be assertive in saying that they do not like something, especially when it comes to how others touch or treat their bodies.

Just because we call sexual behavior normative (normal), this does not mean it is best for the behavior to continue. When you find your young child exploring his or her sexual parts, it is a chance to explain how their body is created by God, that they are fearfully and wonderfully made, and that these special parts of their bodies are to be treated with special honor, which includes not exposing themselves to others (1 Corinthians 12:23). We shared with our children that since the vulva and penis are special parts of your body, they are to be treated with respect, and so we do not play with them like toys. The primary directive we give parents is to have a calm response when they find their children exploring. Take this as an opportunity to gently teach. Any shaming responses, "Don't touch that," "You should never do that," or "That is a no-no!" can send a message to your child that their body is the "no-no" and that having sexual sensations is a bad thing or something to be hidden. Rather, explain God's view and give your direction. You will most likely have to have this conversation multiple times through the years.

Prepare Your Heart for the Talk

When you do talk about sex, check your anxiety level and work through that in order to give your children open, honest, and helpful direction. For many reasons, sexuality brings up a lot of anxiety for parents. Get whatever help and support you need. Also, there may be parts of your conversation that become frustrating, especially if they are older. Remember, fathers (and mothers), "Do not exasperate your children" (Ephesians 6:4). Speak with love (Ephesians 4:15), be frank and direct (Lev 19:17), and open wide your heart (2 Corinthians 6:13). Don't use the Bible to beat God's rules into their head or to condemn your child's thoughts or actions. Teach. Explain. Teach again. With great patience and careful instruction (2 Timothy 4:2).

One of the other things to look at is how you feel about your child being a sexual being. They are, in case you didn't notice. Being a sexual being does not just start when they get married. Each person is a sexual being by the very nature of their physiology—from the moment the fetus begins to develop male and female characteristics during the first few weeks of life in the womb.

As you prepare to talk with your child, check some things about how you have interacted with your child around sexuality up to this point. If you have seen your child touching themselves, how have you reacted? When your child did something that seemed sexual in nature to you, did you ever respond in a way that could have been (or was) rejecting, dismissive, shaming, or ridiculing?

Also, as you read the rest of this chapter, you may realize that you have missed having some of these talks when your children were younger. If they are now a preteen or teen and this is the first time you will be talking, they may have already gotten a message that sex is a taboo subject. If this is your story, your child may have a rather dismissive response, an "I already know that" response. This may be the time to be open with your own discomfort talking about sex and why you possibly delayed having this conversation. This may be a good time to share some of your own story.

Lastly, for married parents preparing to talk with their children about sex, there is often a question about whether their own sexual relationship might have a negative influence on their children. Parents express concerns and questions about how much touch, affection, and kissing they should do in front of their children and whether the kids should know their parents have sex. Also, if intimacy in your marriage is not going well, is there any kind of message your child may be receiving, however subtly? Many adults share memories of hearing arguments between their parents about sex, seeing their mother push away their father's touch, or their father never touching their mom. On the other hand, children, as they age, will say that when they saw their parents engage in affection, it made them feel secure and safe. Even light flirtatious banter or touch between parents for many children is often viewed as positive and loving (even though they will say "ewww"). If you are married, talk about this together as parents; what are your views on the touch between you, how are you feeling it is going between you sexually, and is there anything you'd like to address between you first before talking with your child?

Explaining Anatomy to Children

Parents often have questions about how to talk to their children about sex, and it may help to start by asking yourself how well you know the sexual anatomy. Do you know where the female urethra is? Do you know where the clitoris is? Do you know the structure of the penis? Or what connects the scrotum and the penis and how the sperm gets to the egg? Do your own crash course, not only to make sure you explain correctly, but also so that you deal with your own discomfort.

So how do you explain physiology to children? And what level of detail is appropriate for what ages? We have included a whole chapter, Sexual Anatomy 101, that describes how the vulva, penis, and scrotum are built. You can definitely use the diagrams in this chapter for your child, but these detailed descriptions would be better suited for an older teenager. For younger children, we recommend using books like *God's Design for Sex* (by Carolyn Nystrom and Brenna and Stan Jones) that have tasteful, child-friendly pictures to explain God's plan. Dr. Shelley Metten's *I'm a Girl and I'm a Boy* books have animated pictures and simple anatomy diagrams. At a basic level, when a child is three or four, we recommend explaining how boys and girls are different anatomically and how babies grow within a mom until they are born.

When your child is somewhat older (perhaps six to nine years old) and you are ready to explain to your child how babies are made (see below The Birds and The Bees: The Talk), it will be important to explain about the penis and scrotum and how they operate: what the parts of the penis are, how urine comes out of the penis, where sperm is made, how it travels to the penis, and how during sex the penis enters the vagina and deposits sperm. Also explain about the vagina, the vulva, and the breasts: what the different parts of the vulva are (lips, clitoris, vaginal opening, urethra); where urine exits the female body; how breasts develop; and how an egg travels from the ovaries to the uterus, how the sperm enters the body during sex, travels to the egg, and then how the egg implants into the female body. Making it normal to talk so specifically about their bodies and how sex happens is one way to communicate how good God's creation is and to validate their questions and wonderings.

The Birds and the Bees: The Talk

As we mentioned earlier, we recommend starting to talk with your children when they are young. We recommend using a set of books (*God's Design for Sex* series). When our children were three, four, and five, we used the pictures and reading of the first book to explain how wonderfully God made the body and the ways God made boys and girls different. By early grade school (first grade), we shared the specific details about how babies are made in the plan of God, explaining about how a man and woman who love God get married, and then they have sex and the penis enters the vagina. We knew that they were going to hear all kinds of details from older kids at school, on the playground, in the bathroom, and on the field. We knew our kids needed to have an accurate description that gave honor to God. These conversations were filled with some curious, sometimes embarrassed questions and laughter. I (Tim) spoke initially with the boys and Jennifer spoke with our daughter. And then we would send them to the opposite parent to have a follow-up talk over ice cream to see if they had any other questions. We continued through the years to have increasingly more detailed conversations as they matured.

Specifically, in that conversation between years six and nine, make sure to explain the anatomy as explained above and then explain the process, how...

- the testicles make sperm and send it to the penis.
- when erect during intercourse, the penis enters the vagina and sends the sperm into the vagina.
- the sperm might then swim to reach the egg and fertilize it while

the egg is in the female fallopian tubes, eventually coming to rest in the uterus.

- the baby grows within the mother's uterus for nine months and then is born, coming out through the vagina.

This simple explanation might lead to more questions. You can explain that when a man and woman love each other and are married, they have sex (yes, we recommend you tell them mommy and daddy have sex) and that sometimes having sex results in having a baby, sometimes it does not, but that sex is enjoyable. Your children need to hear from you how good and pleasurable sex is and that God made it that way. Ultimately, make sure that this is just the first of many conversations.

Great Conversations

As your children age, as they go from elementary school into middle school, most likely, they will give you all kinds of openings to talk about sexuality that you don't want to miss. Listen to their music. Talk about the meaning of the lyrics. These can be some amazing opportunities to have some great conversations. When scenes happen during their television shows or in a movie, take the time to discuss their thoughts. If they are reading books that contain a romantic relationship or that refer to some level of a physical relationship, it's important that parents know the content of these books and have healthy conversations with their child. Before the smartphone, when our children had iPods, we were involved with helping them choose the music they added by printing out and discussing the lyrics before they put it on their device. And when our kids received a list of books recommended by a teacher, we looked through them together and realized together that their teachers could have done a much better job of vetting the content. You can have wonderful talks with your children about sex, sexuality, and all the things that lead up to it just by spending some time in their world. Explore their world with them and let the things they are involved in become an opportunity for great conversations.

Sexuality and the Physical Body: Late Elementary School through the Teen Years

Childhood Weight. There are a number of ways that family, parents, grandparents, and caregivers can negatively and positively affect how a child views sex. An important issue that may not seem sexual is how a family talks about the body. When parents make negative comments in front of their child about their own bodies, or about how they need to lose weight, a child can pick up a negative message about their own body. When parents disparage their own weight or fitness level, if they practice dieting, use protein powders to bulk up, or if they make negative comments about their own body, their child's body, or other people's bodies, their children are watching and often develop their own discontent with their bodies.

Check a few things. Do you ask your children if an outfit makes you look fat? Do your children hear you making comments about what you can and cannot eat due to your latest diet or fitness plan? Do you tell your kids that they need to lose weight and that they probably should not eat that? Do your children hear you making negative comments about others' bodies (someone's lack of muscles, the amount of fat on their bodies, the size of someone's breasts)? It may be hard to think that some of these things could be negative. It's good to be fit and trim, right? However, the point here is that your children are watching you and hearing you. They see what you are doing with your own body. If you have issues with your own body image, this will not only affect how they view their own bodies and others' bodies, but it will affect their growing sexuality. If you make negative, demeaning, or derogatory comments about other people's bodies, this can affect how your child views their own body, how they think about others, and what they think constitutes attractiveness. They hear your negative words when they look at themselves in the mirror, even if you never directed those comments to them. Those kinds of responses can lead to eating disorders, a covering up of the body, feelings of shame in connection to their body, self-harm, and sexual acting out. Research shows that negative body image is associated with a negative view of oneself as a sexual person, out-of-control sexual behavior, and low satisfaction in the sexual relationship in marriage. So start to pay attention to how you speak about and interact around your own body, your child's body, and other people's bodies.

Puberty. In Their Own Words:

"I don't even remember talking about what was going to happen in my body. My sister showed me how to put a tampon in."

"There just wasn't any response. I had to figure it out on my own. When I started my period, I told my mom and she was like, 'Tell your sister. Your sister will help you.' She probably felt like we'd relate more or something. But my mom always came across just way too busy to be involved."

"I went and got my own bra by myself. I just did everything by myself."

"When I first started and I was thirteen, I was at my grandmother's. And I didn't tell anybody. I was a late bloomer. When I got home my mom wanted to know where all my underwear had gone, and I said I had started my period. And she said, 'You know where the pads are in the back.' And that was the extent."

These are quotes from women involved in a research study on women's experiences of shame and sexuality. They are perfect examples of common experiences that both boys and girls have with their family members around puberty and their changing bodies. Some families talk about puberty and the changes in the maturing body. Many families just rely on what the school program will teach. Some parents will say, "How was it?" after their child sees the puberty video at school, and then ask, "Do you have any questions?" But then, after that, no other conversation happens. Other families have no conversation at all.

When parents do not involve themselves during this time of great change in the physical body of their child, it can be such a missed opportunity for closeness. It can also be a missed opportunity for creating confidence in the body God has given them. Boys need to know about how their testicles and penis are changing. They need to discuss erection and wet dreams. They need to be able to share their fears about the hair or lack of hair on their body, their muscles or lack of muscles. Girls need to be able to talk about their breasts and what bras to wear. They need to be able to share if they feel insecure about the size of their breasts as they grow. They need to have someone show them how tampons and pads work. And the one these young girls and boys need to have these conversations with is their parent. Yes, they might act uncomfortable with you when you try, but Mom, Dad, don't allow your own discomfort to keep you from having an open conversation with them. Yes, they saw it all in the video. That doesn't mean your part is over. Share what you remember of your own concerns or questions at that age. Talk about your own insecurities. Tell them what kinds of things are happening to their body, and what some of your worries or wonderings were when they were happening to you. This is an incredible opportunity to talk openly and honestly about the body in a way that lets them know that it's normal and doesn't have to be avoided.

Discussing Sexual Arousal and Self-Touch

Why would you teach your child about arousal? Won't that make them want to explore and create arousal? Won't that lead to masturbation and sex? These are the fears that many parents express. And they bring up such a valid point. Should a parent just teach physiology (how babies are made and puberty), or should they also teach their child what exactly is happening when they touch themselves or feel arousal? We recommend that you teach both. If you don't, they are going to hear it from an older child or from the Internet. Or, because you don't talk openly about it with them, they are going to feel like everything about that subject and that part of their body is off limits and taboo.

We explain how arousal happens in chapter eight, *Sexual Anatomy 101*. This is the part of explaining sex to your child that every parent wants to avoid. And the vast majority do. Parents might teach how babies are made, but it is extremely rare to find a parent who explains arousal. It is just too uncomfortable and embarrassing. However, it is critical that you do a good job explaining what is happening to them physiologically, especially as kids approach puberty, and definitely throughout puberty and after. They are wondering, and who is more suited to explain this than their parent? Explain the blood flow, explain the tingling and throbbing. Explain how wet dreams happen. How arousal happens during sexual dreams. Make sure you understand what is happening so that you can explain it. Read the section on arousal in chapter eight. And then explain God's plan on what to do with those sensations. Teach them how to apply their spiritual beliefs to their bodily sensations. As they mature, talk openly about self-touch and masturbation. Read the chapter on masturbation together. Parents, when they are emotionally and physically mature enough, and when you have done some good work around your own purity, share with your child your own convictions and what has helped you get there.

Final Review: The Dos and Don'ts

Remember that a part of your child developing a healthy self-esteem is having a healthy view of their self as a sexual person. Parents need to validate how their child expresses themselves even when they are interested in things that are not considered typical for their gender. This is true for girls in the area of what they want to play with when they are young (dolls vs. trucks), and who they want to be when they grow up (nurses vs. doctors, engineers vs. social workers). This is also true for boys in what kinds of toys and activities they enjoy (if they like sparkly things and dancing, rather than cops and robbers and baseball) and what careers they want to follow (the arts and nursing vs. accounting and business). As a society and as parents, we can have such strict rules around gender that it can harm our children.

Parents also need to validate their child's possession of genitals and normalize their sexual exploration, while teaching them God's view of both their bodies and sex. Sexual problems develop from childhood to adulthood when negative responses to sexuality become connected with someone's self-esteem, when their sexual exploration is shamed, or when it is taboo to speak about sex in the family. One of the best antidotes is to talk openly, spiritually, concretely, and in a matter-of-fact way about sexual topics.

So work at being as comfortable as possible talking with your child about sex. In the midst of those conversations, here are some overall dos and don'ts. Don't shame or punish them for sexual self-touch. If they act out sexually, don't reject them. Jesus didn't. Teach. Pray. Be humble. Establish healthy boundaries. But don't reject them or ridicule them. If something happens to them, if they have been touched by someone in a way that is violating, do not dismiss them. Do not blame them. Support them and get input on how to respond. Remember, it was extremely hard for them to come and tell you. Make sure to tell them you are glad they did.

Do show physical affection in your family. Give realistic, honest explanations of sexual sensations and feelings. Model godly sexual relationships. Do talk openly, concretely, and matter-of-factly. This is an opportunity to show your child the very character of God. Do have ongoing discussions with your child. As they mature, do share your own challenges. Do hug them. And hug them some more. And in these ways, model the very heart of God.

CHAPTER 16

FOR SINGLE AND MARRIED
PARENTS—YOUR EXAMPLE
OF SEXUALITY

You are a married parent and you are wanting to have healthy conversations with your kids about sex, but there are some issues in your marriage and in how you both handle parenting that might be making that challenging.

You are a single parent and you hope to raise your child in a way that both guards and guides their sexuality, but you have some doubts about how to do that as a single parent.

These kinds of challenges might have brought you to this book. This chapter is in more of a Q & A format. These are real questions from parents like you. Hopefully, the answers will be helpful as you navigate these issues. This chapter is also a living document. With future editions, we hope to include even more questions from you. So send us your questions. We would love to hear from you. And now, let's look at what parents like you are asking.

For Married Parents: Your Sexual Relationship

How do we talk to our kids about sex when this area is not going well in our marriage?

This is an incredibly important question. The single most important factor in raising children with a healthy, godly view of sexuality is to work on your own marital sexual relationship. But, to be honest, most people would rather skip the work on their own relationship and move straight into helping their children! This appears to be reflected in the difference in how married folks responded and continue to respond to our two books on sex. Seeing *The Art of Intimate Marriage* title, they glance briefly and move on. They might be thinking, *"There are a lot of marriage books out there. We've already heard a lot of different teaching through the years on what our marital sexual relationship is supposed to be like. Do we really want to look at another book (one that exposes all our most uncomfortable hang ups)? Besides, things probably won't really change."* But then these individuals glance at *Redeemed Sexuality*, see that it is a book about sex for teens, singles, and students and immediately purchase five copies. It is good they are buying the book; however, the single greatest thing we would tell that married individual or couple is to read *The Art of Intimate Marriage* first. The best way to influence your children's sexuality is to work on yours.

But what if you are in a situation where you spouse has not given you any indication he/she is willing to work on things? Yes, this can be very discouraging. But one person can start a revolution, even in a marriage. Go ahead and do the work on yourself, pray for your partner, and see what happens. Your commitment to your own work will have a profound impact on how you speak with your child. Many of the exercises found in this book will still apply. Get your own deep convictions and renew your understanding of Scripture. Talk with someone you trust about what you are learning. Then, when you get with your child, have a genuine talk. Share your own process, how much you have learned as you have done your own work. And then share with them God's plan. His Word will never come back void.

We are newly married and it is a second marriage for both of us. Our kids are old enough to be fully aware we are having sex. Should we be discussing this in some way?

This is a very real situation, not only for remarried parents but for all parents. It is very healthy for children to know that their parents are having sex, especially when this is genuinely shared without more detail than your children are seeking. Sometimes children, especially older children, may catch a glimpse (through an unlocked door) or even hear noises that seem to say you are engaging sexually. And if they are older, most likely they know you are having sex. Having honest conversations about it can go a long way toward conveying that it is OK to ask questions and talk about sex in general.

However, with blended families that are recently married, there may be additional difficulties if children or teens are not yet resolved about the divorce or about their parent being married to someone else. Open up the doors and have the conversation. When you sense your kids are fully aware, it is important to just bring it out into the open. They may not want to discuss it at all, but send a message that you are willing to talk. We also recommend reading *The Smart Step-Family* by Ron Deal.

We have a good sexual relationship, but how much should our children know about what we do sexually?

Most kids do not want to know much about what you are doing sexually. In fact, sharing the specifics could create some overly loose boundaries that can be unhealthy. This is especially true when things are not going well. Parents who share negative details about their sex lives, especially when this is communicated in resentment and anger, create some serious challenges for their children. However, it is vital that parents, in appropriate ways, share with their children that sex is enjoyable and part of the joy of marriage. If you have married children, you may talk more specifically about things that you as a couple mutually agree to share. Do remember that your married kids may not want too many pictures in their heads.

My spouse is uncomfortable with us doing certain kinds of things in front of our kids? What do we do about that? **and** *My husband doesn't like to show affection openly, especially in front of our kids. So, they don't think we even have sex. How should I handle it?*

This is a common difference between parents. Some individuals like to kiss in front of their kids and some do not. Some will pat their spouse's butt in view of their children. Others feel angry if their spouse does that. For some, even these light or playful interactions feel wrong. Culture and background play a lot into these kinds of feelings and choices. The most important thing is to talk about this together and to genuinely listen to what concerns both of you have. Validate those concerns (for more on Validation, see *The Art of Intimate Marriage*, chapter three, four, and five). Listen and ask questions. Review the chapter on family background (chapter two) to explore what might be affecting these feelings.

Do remember that engaging in these kinds of light, affectionate, intimate touches as a married couple can be very healthy for children to see. However, forcing this kind of touch in front of the children when a spouse is not comfortable can cause damage both to your marriage and to your children's view of sexuality. Talk with those you are close to and come up with how to be sensitive to each other while also embracing the beauty of a loving, affectionate marital relationship and the positive impact that can have on children.

"My spouse and I have very different thoughts about things like masturbation. What should we do when talking to our kids?"

This topic brings up strong responses. The spouse who approves of masturbation believes their reasons are strong. The spouse that disapproves also has strong reasons. Both parents may be very reactive about the entire subject. It may bring up some dynamics in your own relationship that need to be worked through. If you are concerned that you are having an out-of-proportion response to how strongly you feel about masturbation, this can be a good chance to explore why. Convictions are important. The way we convey them might expose some needs we ourselves have.

A healthy conversation with your kids about masturbation should occur in the context of an overall open conversation about sex. Some children begin touching themselves much younger. Teaching body awareness and God's plan for sex might be the place to start. For older children, talking about the specifics of masturbation would probably happen either before or during puberty when your child is experiencing an increase in hormones that can lead to an increase in touching themselves. Whatever your circumstances, even if you disagree, you could try discussing some open-ended questions with your children such as these:

"There are many different views of masturbation whether it is
    wrong or healthy? What do you think?"

"What does the Bible say about sexuality that might be
    helpful? How do you think these scriptures might apply to
    masturbation?"

Another suggestion would be to read Save Yourself (chapter twelve). If your child is a teenager, you could read the chapter together and then discuss it. Avoid the lectures but share your own challenges and convictions. Be real. And then let the truth of God's Word do the work. "The Counselor...will convict" (John 16:8). Let the Spirit do the work as you share the truth.

For Single Parents: Your Example in Sexuality

I'm a single mom. I don't even know where to begin with how I should talk with my kids about sex and *How do I teach my 3-year old son about sex, as a single mom?*

There are some unique challenges that come with single parenting and talking with kids about sex. Some single parents carry a lot of guilt for their sexual choices. Others have not had positive experiences in previous relationships or marriages. Others are concerned that even bringing up the subject might lead their kid to engaging in sex before they are married. Also, if a parent is the opposite gender of their child, the question arises, should I even be the one to have that talk. And when I do, how do I do it?

Without being repetitive, we would recommend that you do your own exploration of your views on sex by reading this entire book. After you have done your own work, if they are old enough, read portions of this book together with your child. If they are younger, we recommend the series of books *God's Design for Sex*. If they are preschool age, start with the first book. Go out together somewhere and talk about it. You may be doing some of your own growing in this area while you are teaching your child, and there is nothing wrong with that. Humility is one of the best teachers. Also, sharing about the questions you had at their ages can send a message to your kid that it is OK to wonder and question and ask.

I had sex before I was married. How can I call my kid to wait? I feel like a hypocrite and I've blown it so much in my sexual choices in life. Where do I begin explaining things to my kids?

The Old Testament is full of examples that Paul says we should learn from. "Now these things occurred as examples to keep us from setting our hearts on evil things as they did" (1 Corinthians 10:6). Paul himself had committed some very serious sins against Christians, imprisoning them and giving approval to their deaths (Acts 8:1). So how did Paul view his past sin? "For I am the least of the apostles and do not even deserve to be called an apostle, because I persecuted the church of God. But by the grace of God I am what I am, and his grace to me was not without effect. No, I worked harder than all of them—yet not I, but the grace of God that was with me" (1 Corinthians 15:9-10). Our children need a living example of a balanced view of our sin and God's grace, so that they can find the same balance in their lives. We encourage you to reflect both the gravity of your past sexual sin and the impact that grace has had on your life.

Look at what Paul says about the rest of us: "Do not be deceived: Neither the sexually immoral nor idolaters nor adulterers nor men who have sex with men nor thieves nor the greedy nor drunkards nor slanderers nor swindlers will inherit the kingdom of God. And that is what some of you were. But you were washed, you were sanctified, you were justified in the name of the Lord Jesus Christ and by the Spirit of our God." (Romans 6:9-11).

Notice what he includes in this list of sin. Yes, he includes sexual sin and a host of other sins, but he also lists idolatry, greed, and slander. We don't tend to take those as seriously, yet Paul lets us know that whatever our background is, we all commit these sins and are in desperate need of being washed—and that is what each disciple is. Washed. So when you speak with your child, share how wonderful it is to be washed of wrong, to be justified even though you had sinned. And then share God's plan. As you speak, you can share the painful consequences of whatever sins you committed and then you can share the wonder of the grace that God has shown you.

I'm a single dad with daughters. How should I teach my girls about how God wants them to live sexually?

There are a number of different ways a single dad can go about this. For some single parents who have children of the opposite gender, they are able to have someone they trust, someone their child knows, have these talks with them. However, some parents have the kind of relationship where they themselves can have this conversation with their child. The principle thing is to make it OK to talk about it, whether with you or a trusted friend. Our cultures can make it particularly difficult, though, for men to talk with their daughters about sex. It is vital for young girls to know that they can talk with their dads. Read parts of this book together and ask them their thoughts. However, talking in detail about their own bodies can be particularly uncomfortable for young girls and their embarrassment may be stronger if the conversation is with a man, even a dad they love and trust. Consider teaching them biblically about sex and then allow them to have further talks with a mother of a friend they feel close to about things particular to being girls. It can be quite beneficial for young girls to hear their father's perspective on God's plan for sex and it can also give them a chance to speak with another woman who can relate in unique ways.

I had a lot of negative experiences in my past in sexuality and have avoided talking about this with my kids for fear they could make some wrong choices.

As parents, part of our job is to protect our children and to train them in the way they should go (Proverbs 22:6). However, sometimes our fears can dictate how we go about doing that. Parenting out of fear can make discerning God's will difficult. It is a common fear that if a child has knowledge of something, that means they will go engage in it. There is some truth to that. "I would not have known what sin was had it not been for the law. For I would not have known what coveting really was if the law had not said, 'You shall not covet.' But sin, seizing the opportunity afforded by the commandment, produced in me every kind of coveting" (Romans 7:7-8).

Our children have a sinful nature, and knowing what sin is can lead to sinning. However, look at the example of God. He is the perfect Father, and He lays His commands before each of us and calls us to choose life. He did this from the very beginning. And Adam and Eve chose to sin. Remember, Satan's power is in keeping things in the dark. The power of

God is that He is light. Explaining sin to our children, in age appropriate ways and times, and then showing them the light of God in His Word is parenting as our Father parents. At the age appropriate time (as they approach or are through puberty and are growing in emotional maturity), you could tell your child about the negative experiences, share with them what the consequences were that you experienced in connection to those choices, and then, as we mentioned above, teach them the beauty of God's plan for sex. This can hopefully lead your child to a fuller understanding of why God would put such clear boundaries around sex and what the benefits would be in trusting God in their sexual choices.

Parents, we leave you with this scripture: "God gently leads those that have young" (Isaiah 40:11). He understands, like no other, the challenges of parenting and His hands are gentle on us as we navigate these waters.

CHAPTER 17

TOUCHY TOPICS:
MORE CONVERSATIONS

In today's world, when kids reach middle school and high school, many of them have heard quite a bit about sex. They might not understand it all, but they are hearing it. They are hearing about teenagers getting pregnant. They are hearing about blow jobs, or they might even be the recipient of an offer to receive one. They are hearing that oral sex is okay and that it is not actually having sex. "You can still be a virgin and have oral sex" is the common view. They are hearing and talking about transgender individuals, about the gay and lesbian community (LGBT), and many other forms of alternative sexuality (think *Fifty Shades of Grey*—and if you do not know about this movie, we can promise you, most likely your teenagers do).

Parents (or spiritual mentors) can feel very unsure how to address these topics; however, the best approach is an honest and direct conversation. Talk openly without condemnation about their thoughts when teens or someone that is not married gets pregnant. Ask them questions and let them ask questions. Give honest, direct answers. As your children reach middle school and high school, check in with them about what is happening at their schools and among their fellow students. If you read the chapter *What's a Teen to Do?*, you will see that most of these teens were hearing about oral and anal sex and blow jobs beginning in middle school. We recommend you read this chapter together and ask them if any of these things are similar to their experiences.

Let's consider some of the touchy questions we have been asked. These, in addition to what you learned in previous chapters, will help you open up important and relevant conversations.

"How do we talk about LGBT issues?"

Our number one answer: Read *Caring Beyond the Margins* by Guy Hammond. Read it together with your child, chapter by chapter, and have some great conversations. Chapter seven of this book, *Sexual Identity Development*, should prove helpful as well. Then after you have read those together, prayerfully your ears and eyes will be open for opportunities to talk. You'll find the opportunities may come often. For instance, you can ask them their thoughts about the various stories in the news and the content of TV shows and movies they like to watch. Better yet, you can sit and watch them together and discuss them afterwards. Since your kids are hearing and reading about many alternate sexual practices, ask the Spirit to open up times for life-giving talks about these sensitive topics. Always remember the kindness and patience of God as you talk about LGBT concerns with your kids. Remember that if you are comfortable and curious, they will be more likely to want to talk.

"Should you discipline your kids if you discover them viewing porn or masturbating? If so, how?" and *"We have found searches on sexual topics on our computer that our kids have done. What do we do? Should we discipline them?"*

Glad you asked. The word discipline is important in these questions. "The Lord disciplines those he loves" (Hebrews 12:6). The word for discipline here is *paideuo*, which means train, educate, correct, chastise. You love your children. You want to help guide them. You know there are certain things they cannot be allowed to do, both because they are harmful for them and because of the importance of obedience to God. Also, there might be things they engage in (i.e., pornography) that you do not want in your home. Each of the words that define discipline, therefore, applies to the question above. If you train them, you are disciplining them. Training is vital. But training is most effective when it considers your child's thoughts and motivation. You will need to draw your kids out in order to find out what exactly it is that needs to be trained. Their use of masturbation and pornography may have any number of motivations. Give them shelter and mercy so that they feel safe enough to be real. Parents can sometimes use consequences but fail to take the time to get to the heart of the issue or to help their kids learn good life skills. Take the time to train and educate. After you've listened well, help them to understand the incredible damage of pornography, both to themselves and to those who are in those pictures and videos. If your convictions come from your own personal exposure or sin, this is a great opportunity to share. You can see how this will be more successful if it is one part of a bigger conversation about good sexual habits and what to do with the many pictures flooding their view and the feelings of arousal that might be coursing through them. Do some good training on physiology using the materials in this book. And train them in the Scriptures.

When it comes to correction, use the Word and do so with patience and care. "Correct, rebuke, and encourage, with great patience and careful instruction" (2 Timothy 4:2). We are called as parents to correct their course. However, the tone you use will be vital. Another part of the definition of discipline, chastisement (rebuke would be a more current term), has more to do with consequences and punishment. We do not recommend any discipline or punishment for masturbation. Your patient teaching and explaining, without shaming, are very needed but giving consequences for masturbation will not bring about the benefit you are looking for.

Rebuke or parental discipline is needed when a child is at a fork in the road that could either take them onto the path of life or a onto a destructive course. This calls for a parent to set firm boundaries for their child and implement consequences if they break those boundaries. Discovering that your child habitually uses pornography (which is different from a teen being exposed to pornography) requires parental love with healthy, firm guidelines. That may mean taking away and/or putting serious restrictions on all electronic devices.

Regardless of whether your child has these struggles or not, to guide their course, we recommend that all electronics (TVs, computers, handheld devices, etc.) are kept out of the bedrooms and that phones are locked down at bedtime. Consider using programs like Safe Eyes and Covenant Eyes to safeguard your family and your home. However, the best guardian is prayer, the Holy Spirit, and planting the Word of God in their hearts—not just in the area of sexuality, but in all areas.

"One of our kids walked in on us while having sex. What do we do?"

Many of us have stories of hearing and seeing things that happened with our own parents. If it hasn't already, it very likely will happen at some point in your children's upbringing. Let us share a story. One of our kids as a teenager told us they heard some things as they were going to bed. I, Jennifer, asked, with a slight smile, "What did you do?" and my kid said, "I put in my ear plugs." "Gotcha," with a nod, was my answer. We both laughed and that was the end of it. If your child walks in on you, after they have left (probably running), or when they come and tell you, sit down with them and ask if they have any questions. It's healthy for kids to know their parents have sex. However, just knowing is probably enough details. If they are willing, have an open conversation about how they feel about walking in on you or overhearing something. And then consider if you need to invest in locks or teach children to knock.

If my son is addicted to porn and masturbation, how should we as parents handle talking about it? Should I as a mom be involved at all?"

These are such tough things. To answer the last part of this question, in general there are different parts that each parent can bring to these conversations. Remember, dad can also provide—and moms can also add—a different dimension for their sons. So talk about it together as a couple and pray that God will use each of you to be of benefit to your child.

The use of pornography and masturbation are so very damaging, and knowing what to do can be challenging. First of all, it may be helpful to know the difference between use and addiction. We've discussed this somewhat in chapter eleven and chapter fifteen. So why is the distinction between use and addiction important? On a spiritual level, whether something has reached an addiction level or not doesn't change that it could be wrong. However, if something has gotten to a level of use where someone is trying to stop and feels like they can't (which can happen quickly with pornography), then the type of help they need might be different. There are many different types of addiction (i.e., food, drugs, alcohol, gambling, sex, etc.) but they all have certain similarities:

- Multiple unsuccessful tries to quit
- Spending a lot of time doing it or plotting to do it
- Diving in even when there are damaging consequences both to the individual and to those around them
- Needing to do more and more in order to get the desired effect
- Experiencing irritation, anxiety, and agitation when unable to or having to delay being able to do it

So a behavior may be compulsive, where the desire to masturbate or do pornography has increased in frequency and has become very hard to resist, but may not yet be an addiction. Note: Do be careful about using the word addiction quickly or lightly with teens.

As you seek to keep your child safe and reduce the danger they face, do remember these scriptures:

"Each person is tempted when they are dragged away by their own evil desire and enticed. Then, after desire has conceived, it gives birth to sin; and sin, when it is full-grown, gives birth to death."

JAMES 1:14-15

"See to it, brothers and sisters, that none of you has a sinful, unbelieving heart that turns away from the living God. But encourage one another daily, as long as it is called 'Today,' so that none of you may be hardened by sin's deceitfulness."

HEBREWS 3:12-13

"Opponents must be gently instructed, in the hope that God will grant them repentance leading them to a knowledge of the truth, and that they will come to their senses and escape from the trap of the devil, who has taken them captive to do his will."

2 TIMOTHY 2:25-26

What do we learn here? And how would we apply this to a child who might be developing some compulsive habits? Let's focus on a few things and how you can use them with your child. First, pay attention to the desire and enticement. These are the pulls towards a behavior, the temptations. We often just deal with the full-grown sin and fail to work at the level of enticement (see Jennifer's addiction website theransomedjourney.com for more). However, we recommend helping your child (or yourself, if it also applies to you) to begin to recognize what is drawing them. For teens, the draw may be that they have a hard time asking questions they have about sex; it could be connected to wanting to go along with the crowd; it may have become a stress reducer; or it may make them feel wanted and attractive. Take the time to find out.

Secondly, recognize that encouragement and gentle instruction can help keep your teen's heart from becoming hard and even help them have victory over these dangers and these pulls. Make sure you're giving lots of encouragement in the midst of the prayer, worry, distress, and frustration. And when you do speak with them, be gentle.

Lastly, remember who the enemy is. It is not your teen and what they are doing. When we get deeply entrenched in any sin, it becomes a trap and we become captive. Satan is the entrapper. We need to remember this when dealing with any sin. Remember, it is difficult sometimes for teenagers to come to their senses because their senses are still developing. Their prefrontal cortex—that planning, thinking, evaluating part of their brain—will not fully mature until they are in their mid-twenties. So for now, when they feel guilty, they might hide. When they feel shame, they might shut down or get defensive. If your child has a flat face when you talk with them about these kinds of things, take care to not automatically interpret that flat face as a lack of remorse or a lack of taking something seriously. Often that lack of expression is more a reflection of overwhelming feelings and a very difficult time knowing how to respond to you or what to say. Therefore, remember to hold on to your hope in God, pray that God will work on them to bring about change, put safe boundaries into place, teach and train, and be patient and encouraging.

"How do I answer my child when they ask about oral or anal sex?"

When a child or teen asks a tricky question, one of the best first responses can be, "What a good question. I'm glad you asked it." It may also help to find out where the question is coming from. So draw your child out. "So tell me what you've heard about it so far." As kids get older, they want to know if it's OK to do certain things. To review, we recommend an honest, but not detailed, answer. When our child asked if we engaged in oral sex, this was our response: "God made our bodies and when you are married, any part of your body can touch any part of their body, and any part of their body can touch any part of yours." If your child is older, share with them the *What's Allowed List* found in this book. We do want to emphasize that the first thing to do when your kids ask you one of these sticky questions is to tell them you're glad they asked and that you're impressed with their willingness to bring it up.

Just when we think we've prepared for any question they might ask, our child comes up with something new. A social media we've never heard about. A new sexual practice that kids are experimenting with. When they bring up these topics, one of the most powerful things a parent can do is admit they don't have all the answers Asking your teen for some time can be wise. "Honey, that is a great question. Can I take some time to think about it and get back to you?" So, parents, have these conversations with your children. It is vital that they know that no subject is off limits and that they can speak with you even about the most controversial and volatile of topics.

CONCLUSION

What again is Redeemed Sexuality? You have been with us on a journey. And the hope is that through this journey, you have been able to gain a new experience of sexuality, seeing it as the precious gift that it is. God's Word uniquely allows us to experience sexuality free from distress, harm, or captivity.

We have shared a lot in these pages. With your head now spinning with so many thoughts and scriptures, where would you go from here? You may have read this book straight through in one sitting. We have had people tell us this is exactly what they did. Or you may have carefully read each page, slowly and with meditation, examining each point. You may have read portions, put it down for a while, and read more as the need arose. Our hope and prayer is that you will have a renewed understanding of the power of sexuality for someone who loves and follows Jesus.

God desires for each of us to live out our sexuality in the sunlight. If you'll remember, in Philippians we found a unique term for purity, *eilikrines*, which means when something is so pure it can withstand being judged in the sunlight. Set your heart on the beauty and majesty of God as you pursue standing with Him in the sunlight. "One thing I ask of the Lord, this is what I seek; to dwell in the house of the Lord all the days of my life, to gaze upon the beauty of the Lord, and to see Him in His dwelling place" (Psalm 27:4).

If you are single or not currently married, consider marking the passages in this book that either inspired you or troubled you, and pray about them. Take the scriptures to a mountain top, the ocean cliffs, or your favorite place of retreat and call out to God for wisdom and understanding. He promises to hear you (James 1:5). If you desire marriage, pray and plan for your future and then surrender your hopes and desires to the God who cares for you.

If you are a parent reading this, remember, God has your children in His hands. He gently leads those that have young (Isaiah 40:11). He sees the heart and effort you are putting into your parenting and He will gently lead you.

If you are a college student or teen, you have the opportunity to give God your undivided attention and to be a beacon on a hill. Pursue purity as the incredible privilege it is, and if you fall, look to your Father. "As the eyes of slaves look to the hand of their master, as the eyes of a female slave look to the hand of her mistress, so our eyes look to the LORD our God, till he shows us his mercy" (Psalm 123:2).

So here, at the conclusion of this journey with us, we recommend some steps on what to do after you have read this book.

Number One. Without sounding trite, be in the Word and pray every day. The best route you can take to having the precious sexuality that God intends, free from distress, harm, and captivity, is to get on the road each morning by spending time talking with God and listening to Him.

Number Two. Examine the many scriptures found in this text. "Each man should be fully convinced in his own mind" (Romans 14:5). It is vital that each of us take the time to gain personal convictions from the Scriptures in order to understand what God expects of us in our sexual lives.

Number Three. Spend some time writing out all that stands out to you or talking with a trusted friend about what you gained from reading this book. For instance, you might make a top five list of convictions you want to take away from your first reading.

Number Four. Make a plan.

If you are a parent, start with a plan for yourself. What do you need to work on in living out your own sexuality? Then think through and write out a plan about how you want to guide your child. Get input on your plan and pray about it. Pray again. Then spend special time with your child having life-enriching conversations.

If you are a single, teen, or college student working on your purity, pray about, think through, and write out a specific plan on what you are going to do to live out your sexuality as God desires. Share this with someone you trust. Pray regularly about it. Go back to that person you trust regularly to have them help you stay with your plan or adjust your plan as time goes.

Number Five. The Most Important: KNOW GOD. This goes right along with Number One, but we want to emphasize that in order to live out your life and your sexuality to the fullest, God calls you to a deep knowing of who He is. Get in the Word and know His very character. He is the God that made clothes for Adam and Eve. He is Jesus, whose heart was moved as He saw a widow at her son's funeral. He is the God who created the universe, holds the seas in His hands, and can heal an eyeball in an instant. He takes delight in you (Psalm 149:4). You are God's chosen, His special possession (1 Peter 2:9), and He is longing to be gracious to you and show you compassion (Isaiah 30:18). He is unfailingly patient, unimaginably kind, and immeasurably powerful. Know the God who created you so that you can live out your life in the flesh, bringing glory to Him until you rest in His arms in heaven. It is an amazing thing that as disciples of Jesus, we live in a body inhabited by the Holy Spirit. "Therefore, as dearly loved children, live a life of love" (Ephesians 5:1-2). Amen!

Remember, finally, that God has designed sexuality as something to bring us closer to Him and closer to others. Satan wants to use sexuality to destroy us. If we live our life in submission to God, He can bring about beauty in this area of our lives. He is the master artist. Let Him do His artwork on you. Be the canvas for the display of His glory!

Also by Tim Konzen and Dr. Jennifer Konzen:
The Art of Intimate Marriage:
A Christian Couple's Guide to Sexual Intimacy

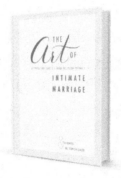

For more resources, please visit www.theartofintimatemarriage.com
and
www.theransomedjourney.com.
The Art of Intimate Marriage and *The Intimate Marriage Cards*
can be ordered online at Amazon.com.